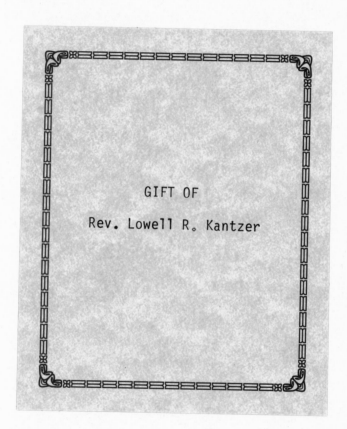

COUNSELING AND REHABILITATING
THE CANCER PATIENT

Publication Number 964

AMERICAN LECTURE SERIES®

A Publication in

The BANNERSTONE DIVISION *of*
AMERICAN LECTURES IN SOCIAL AND REHABILITATION PSYCHOLOGY

Editors of the Series

JOHN G. CULL, Ph.D.
Director, Regional Counselor Training Program
Department of Rehabilitation Counseling
Virginia Commonwealth University
Fishersville, Virginia

and

RICHARD E. HARDY, Ed.D.
Diplomate in Counseling Psychology (ABPP)
Chairman, Department of Rehabilitation Counseling
Virginia Commonwealth University
Richmond, Virginia

The American Lecture Series in Social and Rehabilitation Psychology offers books which are concerned with man's role in his milieu. Emphasis is placed on how this role can be made more effective in a time of social conflict and a deteriorating physical environment. The books are oriented toward descriptions of what future roles should be and are not concerned exclusively with the delineation and definition of contemporary behavior. Contributors are concerned to a considerable extent with prediction through the use of a functional view of man as opposed to a descriptive, anatomical point of view.

Books in this series are written mainly for the professional practitioner; however, academicians will find them of considerable value in both undergraduate and graduate courses in the helping services.

COUNSELING AND

REHABILITATING

THE CANCER PATIENT

RICHARD E. HARDY, Ed.D. *and* **JOHN G. CULL, Ph.D.**

Diplomate in Counseling Psychology (ABPP)

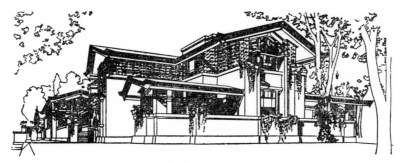

CHARLES C THOMAS · PUBLISHER

Springfield · Illinois · U.S.A.

Published and Distributed Throughout the World by
CHARLES C THOMAS • PUBLISHER
Bannerstone House
301-327 East Lawrence Avenue, Springfield, Illinois, U.S.A.

© *1975, by* CHARLES C THOMAS • PUBLISHER
ISBN 0-398-03297-1
Library of Congress Catalog Card Number: 74-11488

With THOMAS BOOKS *careful attention is given to all details of
manufacturing and design. It is the Publisher's desire to present books
that are satisfactory as to their physical qualities and artistic possibilities
and appropriate for their particular use.* THOMAS BOOKS *will be
true to those laws of quality that assure a good name and good will.*

Printed in the United States of America
W-2

Library of Congress Cataloging in Publication Data
Hardy, Richard E
    Counseling and rehabilitating the cancer patient.

    (American lecture series, publication no. 964. A
publication in the Bannerstone Division of American
lectures in social and rehabilitation psychology)
    1. Cancer patients—Rehabilitation. I. Cull, John
G., joint author. II. Title. [DNLM: 1. Counseling.
2. Neoplasms—Rehabilitation. 3. Patients. QZ200
H271c]
RC262.H29   362.1'9'6994   74-11488
ISBN 0-398-03297-1

To two outstanding rehabilitation practitioners

Mr. Frank O. Birdsall

of Virginia

and

Mr. Charles W. Hoehne

of Texas

The following books have appeared thus far in the Social and Rehabilitation Psychology Series:

MEDICAL AND PSYCHOLOGICAL ASPECTS OF DISABILITY
  A. Beatrix Cobb

DRUG DEPENDENCE AND REHABILITATION APPROACHES
  Richard E. Hardy and John G. Cull

SPECIAL PROBLEMS IN REHABILITATION
  A. Beatrix Cobb

REHABILITATION OF THE DRUG ABUSER WITH DELINQUENT
  BEHAVIOR
  Richard E. Hardy and John G. Cull

COUNSELING HIGH SCHOOL STUDENTS: Special Problems and Approaches
  John G. Cull and Richard E. Hardy

TYPES OF DRUG ABUSERS AND THEIR ABUSES
  John C. Cull and Richard E. Hardy

ALCOHOL ABUSE AND REHABILITATION APPROACHES
  John G. Cull and Richard E. Hardy

ORGANIZATIONAL AND ADMINISTRATION OF DRUG ABUSE
  TREATMENT PROGRAMS: National and International
  John G. Cull and Richard E. Hardy

PSYCHOLOGICAL AND VOCATIONAL REHABILITATION OF THE
  YOUTHFUL DELINQUENT
  Richard E. Hardy and John G. Cull

PROBLEMS OF ADOLESCENTS: Social and Psychological Approaches
  Richard E. Hardy and John G. Cull

PROBLEMS OF DISADVANTAGED AND DEPRIVED YOUTH
  John G. Cull and Richard E. Hardy

FUNDAMENTALS OF JUVENILE CRIMINAL BEHAVIOR AND
  DRUG ABUSE
  John G. Cull and Richard E. Hardy

CONTRIBUTORS

CHARLES ROBERT BLAKE, M.D.: Ophthalmologist at the Thomas-Davis Clinic, Tucson, Arizona; educated at Reed College, Portland, Oregon; University of Washington, Seattle, Washington; Stanford University, Palo Alto, California; University of Southern California, School of Medicine, Los Angeles, California; residency in surgery at the Santa Fe General Hospital, Los Angeles, California; active in pro- Award in 1972 and Community Service Award, Arizona Medical Association, 1973.

A. BEATRIX COBB, Ph.D.: Horn Professor of Psychology Emeritus, Texas Tech University; formerly, Director, Counselor Training Program; head, Medical Psychology Section, University of Texas, M. D. Anderson Hospital and Tumor Institute, and Associate professor, University of Texas Postgraudate School of Medicine; has published widely in various professional journals and has been a contributing author of textbooks in rehabilitation.

JOHN G. CULL, Ph.D.: Professor and Director, Regional Counselor Training Program, Department of Rehabilitation Counseling, Virginia Commonwealth University, Fishersville, Virginia; Adjunct Professor of Psychology and Education, School of General Studies, University of Virginia, Charlottesville, Virginia; technical consultant, Rehabilitation Services Administration, United States Department of Health, Education and Welfare, Washington, D.C.; editor, American Lecture Series in Social and Rehabilitation Psychology, Charles C Thomas, Publisher; lecturer, Medical Department, Woodrow Wilson Rehabilitation Center; formerly, rehabilitation counselor, Texas Rehabilitation Commission; director, Division of Research and Program Development, Virginia State Department of Vocational Rehabilitation; has co-authored and co-

edited *Drug Dependence and Rehabilitation Approaches,
Fundamentals of Criminal Behavior and Correctional
Systems, Rehabilitation of the Drug Abuser With Delinquent
Behavior,* and *Therapeutic Needs of the Family;* and con-
tributed more than sixty publications to the professional
literature in psychology and rehabilitation.

The Late **HARRY H. GARNER, M.D.:** Chairman, Department of
Psychiatry and Behavioral Sciences, University of Health Sci-
ences, The Chicago Medical School; chairman of Department
of Psychiatry and Behavioral Sciences, Mt. Sinai Medical
Center, Chicago; consultant, Hines V.A. Hospital in Chicago,
Oak Forest Hospital, Cook County Hospital, and Illinois State
Psychiatric Institute; Psychiatric Advisory Council, State of
Illinois; Guthiel Von Domarrus Award for contribution to
psychotherapy, A.O.A. Honorary Medical Society; Past Presi-
dent, Illinois Psychiatric Society; Best Teacher Award, Illinois
Psychiatric Institute; formerly, Director of Community Clinics
State of Illinois; attending psychiatrist at Cook County Hospital, Psychopathic Hospital Division; Director of Neuro-
psychiatric Division Branch (Illinois, Indiana, Wisconsin),
Veterans Administration; Clinical Director at Chicago State
Hospital; author of *Psychosomatic Management of the Patient
with Malignancy, Psychotherapy—Confrontation Problem-
solving Technique;* co-editor, *Unfinished Tasks;* wrote chap-
ters in four books on psychiatry; has contributed more than
ninety articles to journals of a professional nature.

RICHARD E. HARDY, Ed.D.: Diplomate in counseling psy-
chology; chairman, Department of Rehabilitation Counseling,
Virginia Commonwealth University, Richmond, Virginia;
technical consultant, United States Department of Health,
Education and Welfare, Rehabilitation Services Administra-
tion, Washington, D.C.; editor, American Lecture Series in
Social and Rehabilitation Psychology, Charles C Thomas,
Publisher; and associate editor, Journal of Voluntary Action
Research; formerly, rehabilitation counselor in Virginia; re-
habilitation advisor, Rehabilitation Services Administration,

United States Department of Health, Education and Welfare, Washington, D.C.; former Chief Psychologist and Supervisor of Professional Training, South Carolina Department of Rehabilitation; and member of the South Carolina State Board of Examiners in Psychology; has coauthored and coedited *Drug Dependence and Rehabilitation Approaches, Fundamentals of Criminal Behavior and Correctional Systems, Rehabilitation of the Durg Abuser with Delinquent Behavior,* and *Therapeutic Needs of the Family;* and contributed more than sixty publications to the professional literature in psychology and rehabilitation.

CECIL O. SAMUELSON, Ph.D.: Professor of Educational Psychology, University of Utah; has been a high school counselor, Assistant State Director of Vocational Rehabilitation and State Director of Guidance Services in Utah; has published numerous articles in rehabilitation and educational journals.

KENT MITCHELL SAMUELSON, M.D.: Received his degree from the University of Utah, interned in surgery at the Orange County Medical Center in California and completed residency in orthopedic surgery at the University of Utah Affiliated Hospitals; has license to practice medicine and surgery in the state of Utah; has several publications in medical journals.

PREFACE

T HE FIRST YEAR of the accelerated federally supported attack against human cancer was 1972. Not only medical researchers and scientists but also all social service workers involved in rehabilitation and counseling with the cancer patient are reaching out in many directions for causes, cures, and methods of providing helping services.

As medical researchers attempt to answer questions such as, "To what extent are viruses involved in causing cancer and what can be done to boost the body's natural defenses against cancer?" rehabilitation and social service workers are attempting to come to grips with improved methods of rehabilitation in terms of vocational evaluation of the cancer victim and general counseling and vocational advisement in terms of realistic goals and objectives. Rehabilitation and social workers are becoming heavily involved with psychotherapeutic care for the cancer patient which requires developing an in-depth feeling for his needs and personal concerns.

A huge problem in all knowledge systems is the facilitation of that knowledge and its broad dissemination. This is true in both physical and social sciences. Dr. A. Hamblin Letton of Atlanta, president of the American Cancer Society, recently stated that existing knowledge could cure two thirds of all Americans who have cancer. This can take place only if all present knowledge is widely known and applied. The rehabilitation and social service professional has a real responsibility in preparing individuals not only for a productive life but also for a death with dignity when this is inevitable. At present, only about one third of cancer patients survive. Certainly during the decade of the 70's much energy, time and funding will go into increasing our knowledge and skills in working with cancer patients. These

xi

funds will come from many sources, the federal government in particular.

We all know so well that cancer as a disease is accompanied by apprehension, anxiety, and a certain amount of discomfort among both the professional persons attempting to help clients and those who are trying to deal on a personal basis with the fact that they have cancer. This book has been developed mainly for the professional practitioner who is concerned with rehabilitation work. It is not a medical textbook but one which should provide very helpful information to various social service professionals including psychologists, rehabilitation counselors, social workers, occupational therapists, and others. It will be of considerable interest however to the layman as he reads about how other persons have gone through various medical, psychological and vocational problems related to the disease.

We wish to thank those who worked with us by making contributions to this material. We are especially indebted to Mrs. Margie Alexy and Mr. James Antonick for their work on the case study materials. Also, we would like to recognize Irvin K. White of Kentucky for his commitment to the vocational rehabilitation of the individual with cancer.

CONTENTS

COUNSELING AND REHABILITATING

THE CANCER PATIENT

Chapter 1

REHABILITATION

AND CANCER

KENT M. SAMUELSON

AND

CECIL O. SAMUELSON

INTRODUCTION

CANCER IS PROBABLY as old as life itself. Signs of it have been found in the bones of ancient animals. It is found today in every kind of living thing—plants, animals, and humans. The Egyptians knew it and treated it with ointments, prayers, and spells; and, no doubt, other peoples in other places and other times had their peculiar remedies, none of which was particularly helpful. Since so little was known about cancer and so little could be done about it and because it so often affected the most intimate parts of the body, it came to be regarded with particular dread as an

3

unmentionable or disgraceful condition (American Cancer Society). But what actually is cancer?

DEFINITION

Cancer may be defined in various ways depending upon who is giving the definition. In a medical sense, cancer is a disease that is characterized by abnormal growth and spread of cells. Cancer typically begins as a "localized" disease. At the start, just one of the tiny cells of the body—or perhaps a few cells— undergoes an unfortunate change; it becomes a malignant cell, cancer. The cancer cell reproduces itself by dividing into two cells which in turn divide, etc. All of the cells that started from the original cancer cell or cells are themselves cancer cells. Thus, the cancer grows (American Cancer Society, 1970).

The person afflicted with cancer or those involved may not think of this relatively simple-sounding biological process. The person so afflicted may define it as a death sentence preceded by untold agony.

PHILOSOPHY

Over the years cancer has been regarded generally as a horrible, incurable disease. Those who became so afflicted were unfortunate and there was not much hope for them. Once the diagnosis was made, it became basically a waiting game—waiting for death which was assumed to be inevitable. Perhaps worst of all was the emptiness of this waiting period which contained little thought for the possibilities of constructive activity on the part of the person caught by this dreadful disease. The posture on the part of all concerned typically was one of hopelessness.

This negative attitude might be expected on the part of the subject and those close to him. What else was there to think in the absence of encouragement from any source? Pondering such an ailment in the atmosphere of its distressing symptoms could bring despair to even the stoutest soul. Healey (1968) says it is easy to understand the lay person's defeatest attitude toward the disease. He learns little about cancer except for the publicity given the fatal cases, reports on the increase in incidence of lung cancer, or the fear tactics used by various cancer societies and insurance agencies. Rarely does he learn of the successes of cancer therapy. But, perhaps the greatest negative influence has come from the attitudes of the individuals in the professional groups to which persons with cancer are exposed. The applicant with cancer who found his way to the vocational rehabilitation office was scarcely reassured by his need to meet the criterion of employability after the rehabilitation service had been rendered. The fears of such an applicant may be further kindled by the need to wait a year or two after the final treatment to make certain that he had been "cured." While from an agency point of view this procedure may appear to reflect sound policy and good judgment on the part of the counselor, it could be devastating to the subject. His morale might waste away at the time when he needed the greatest support; and, from a realistic standpoint, the loss of time waiting for the cure to be verified could not be recovered.

Even some physicians may harbor attitudes out of keeping with the facts about cancer. Healey (1968) reflects this possibility concerning physicians in these words:

> Unfortunately, however, the practicing physician also maintains a negative attitude toward cancer and the rehabilitation potential of patients afflicted with this disease. This attitude generates from certain deficits in his medical education. The average physician, during his medical training, has very limited exposure to cancer patients, and therefore, is poorly informed about the facts of cancer. His training in rehabilitation procedures is even more limited (p. 23).

The substance of this is to stress the need for improving the attitudes and changing the philosophy of all those concerned in the treatment and care of cancer patients. This is more than a platitudinous call for improvement. There is a substantial basis for a more constructive philosophy toward cancer. While there does not seem to be a cure for cancer at the present time, the outlook is far from discouraging. Again Healey (1968) points out that in the 1920's cancer was considered to be an incurable disease. Today, according to the statistics of the American Cancer

Society, one of every three patients obtains a "clinical cure." Holleb (1970) writing about the cancer cures we have now believes that if every cancer were detected and treated in the early stage the cure rate would be increased to one of every two patients despite the fact that we do not know the cause of cancer. This great achievement is possible with the therapeutic methods which are available today. Improved medical and surgical procedures and especially early diagnosis have served to increase the numbers who have survived a five-year period. Time has brought improvement in the outlook for cancer patients.

From a vocationally rehabilitative point of view, cancer has always presented practical problems. Since the state rehabilitative agency was charged with the ultimate employment of the persons it served, the dull future of the cancer patient did not make him a bright prospect for rehabilitative services. Furthermore, a distinction had to be made between physical restoration services which were primarily for purposes of medical care, and those that were for purposes of vocational rehabilitation. The long-standing concern of the Federal Vocational Rehabilitation Administration for the cancer patient and the need to make the above-mentioned distinction in selecting applicants for rehabilitation services were set forth in the guidelines embraced in the *Administrative Service Series, number 64-6,* of August 8, 1963. In the *Commissioner's Letter, number 68-5,* dated August 29, 1967, further instructions were issued concerning eligibility of cancer patients. Among other helpful directions this letter states, "Accordingly we believe that cancer at all stages may be considered a disability which constitutes a substantial handicap to employment." The effect of this statement is to emphasize that cancer is a qualifying disability for rehabilitation purposes and to encourage the state agencies to look with greater receptiveness at applicants so afflicted. Five years ago the Vocational Rehabilitation Administration and the American Cancer Society as indicated in the *Commissioner's Letter, number 68-11,* November 9, 1967, entered into a cooperative agreement embracing joint efforts that included liaison between the organizations, patient referral, professional education, research and demonstration, public education, and consulting services. These developments indicate substantial movement in the rehabilitation of the cancer-afflicted person. Other agencies, organizations, and concerned individuals are moving toward a more realistic and, at the same time, constructive attitude toward cancer and the person it attacks. The future merits our calm and confident reassurance.

MEDICAL INFORMATION

In discussing cancer there are a number of terms that are used by physicians which warrant a general definition that might be helpful to the counselor. The following list is intended to include only some of the more general terms that might be encountered.*

Cancer—An uncontrolled growth of abnormal cells that have a tendency to invade tissues locally and also spread to distant sites. If untreated, the cancer will usually cause death.

Tumor—An abnormal swelling or enlargement made up of a mass of calls which grow as an independent cluster and serve no useful purpose.

Neoplasm—A tumor.

Malignancy—Cancer.

Benign—Nonmalignant.

Carcinoma—A cancer originating in epithelial (covering) tissue.

Sarcoma—A cancer originating in connective tissues, such as muscle, bone, and cartilage.

Leukemia—Cancer of the blood-forming organs (bone marrow, lymph nodes, spleen), characterized by excessive formation of white blood cells.

Lymphoma—Malignant growths of lymph nodes.

Metastasis—The spread of disease from one part of the body to another by direct extension or through the lymph or blood vessels, carrying the characteristic cells from the

---

* For definitions of those terms not listed, it is suggested that the reader refer to books such as *Dorland's Illustrated Medical Dictionary,* 24th edition, S. B. Saunders Company, Philadelphia, 1965; or Taber's *Cyclopedic Medical Dictionary,* 9th edition, illustrated, F. A. Davis Company, Philadelphia, 1962.

first lesion to a new location in the body. It is applied to secondary tumors arising at a distance from the primary growth.

Biopsy—The removal of a small part of a living tissue for microscopic examination to determine whether cancer cells are present.*

Cancer is usually thought of as a process which starts in one location of the body and then spreads to other sites. The major symptoms experienced by the patient may be due to either the primary or metastatic proliferation, or to the systemic effects caused by the abnormal metabolism of cancerous cells. Often cancer is first discovered when the patient has symptoms from a secondary growth; and it is sometimes the metastatic lesion that is threatening life and produces the major problems. Some patients will present only some of the systemic complaints that are usually seen with cancer—weight loss, weakness, anemia, easy fatigability.

Depending upon its type and location, the cancer will usually cause various nutritional deficiencies to occur in the rest of the body which account for the systemic effects. This may be due to loss of nutrients appropriated by the growing tumor, or lost to malabsorption with tumors involving the digestive system. Special dietary and nutritional care may offset this problem temporarily, but long-term nutritional therapy cannot adequately supply the nutrients lost to the tumor (Mayer, Part 1, 1971).

Nutritional and systemic problems can further be compounded by the various forms of treating the malignancy. Surgery, radiation, and anti-cancer drugs can and frequently do cause problems, such as nausea, vomiting, diarrhea, fluid loss, malabsorption, and hemorrhage, to name a few. Nutritional deficiencies secondary to cancer therapy often respond fairly well to dietary management as opposed to those secondary to the disease itself. In such cases, dietary monitoring and management become an important part of the therapy (Mayer, Part 2, 1971).

---

* Adapted from *Teaching About Cancer,* a publication of the American Cancer Society.

In planning an appropriate rehabilitation program for a patient, the question of prognosis becomes an important consideration. There are many factors which influence a prognosis, such as type and location of the malignancy, the stage or degree of advancement when diagnosed, the availability of appropriate therapy, and the response of the body and tumor to the therapy. The evaluation of the many variables involved in each particular patient is the province of the physician, and the counselor must depend upon him for adequate information on this subject.

Prognosis is often given on the basis of five-year survival rates. This simply represents the number of patients in a given series who have had a specific tumor and treatment and who are alive after five years. The period of five years does not carry special significance regarding the cure of cancer as some believe: figures could just as well be given as four-, or six-year survival rates. There are many investigators who use other methods of reporting survival rates and this information is just as valuable. Of course, the longer the follow-up, the more valuable the study becomes in accurately estimating survival.

Shimkin (1951) reported on a review of the literature on the natural history of untreated cancer and gives survival rates in the form of a coordinate graph with survivals extending up to seven years. A method of computing survival rates for patients with chronic diseases has been published by Lillian Axtell (1963). This is another approach which may be used in dealing with cancer statistics and may be more meaningful than five-year survival rates. The details of these procedures are presented in these references.

Cutler and Heise (1971) published twenty-year survival rates for cancer of the uterus, ovary, colon, rectum, and bladder. Cancer of these organs accounted for 56 percent of all cancers in females and 19 percent of all cancers in males that were reported for their study. The data show an upward trend in survival rates, which although confirming the dreaded nature of cancer, offer an encouraging prospect.

The computation of survival rates constitutes important information about cancer, but such data apply to groups and should not be used as a basis for a decision as to whether a particular person is suited for rehabilitative efforts. The following research summary reflects a constructive way of considering the rehabilitation of the cancer patient:

> No accurate judgment of life expectancy or time for useful activity can be estimated for the cancer patient, in spite of the general tables available. Therefore, it is unrealistic and contrary to the concept of total care to defer rehabilitation attention for a waiting period in order to determine the status of the disease or possibility of its spread. Disability from cancer or its treatment can be considered by the same criteria as are used for a noncancer-related disability. The need for supportive care for the patient with advanced cancer should be stressed.*

As with any disease, the cancer patient's family, friends, and contacts are often concerned about the possibility of their contracting the disease. The big questions are: "Is it hereditary?" and "Is it contagious?" Knowing the answers to these questions would certainly influence the way friends and relatives react to and interact with the patient and his disease. The public has generally been taught that "There is no scientific proof that cancer in humans is contagious or inherited" (American Cancer Society). While this statement is true as far as actual proof is concerned, there are some interesting and provocative reports in the literature which suggest that in the future we may not be able to be quite so dogmatic.

The medical literature contains numerous reports of certain types of cancer occurring in various families much more frequently than would be expected statistically (Li, 1970). While such reports certainly do not prove an hereditary basis for cancer, the incidence of such cases is indeed suggestive. Knudson (1970) in writing "Genetics and Cancer," states, "For most cancers it may be said that heredity plays a role, but clarification of this role is not possible at present."

There has also been considerable interest in the relationship between viruses and cancer. Viruses are minute infectious agents that are generally composed of either DNA or RNA and

---

* *Research Brief of Significant Findings—Rehabilitation of Cancer Patients,* Memorial Hospital fo Cancer and Allied Diseases, New York, New York.

are covered by a protein coat. Viruses have been known for a number of years to cause cancer in animals and viral particles have been shown to be present in some malignancies in man (Henke, 1968). The demonstration of a cause-effect relationship between viruses and some cancers in animals, obviously, does not mean that the same is true for man, but the possibility is worthy of consideration. Considerable investigation is being carried out on this subject and Milt (1969) has written a good review of the problem of viruses and cancer.

Incidence

It appears that cancer is assuming an increasingly important role as a cause of death and disability among people for whom such statistics are kept. Cancer is found among all peoples who have been studied, although some forms of cancer appear to be more common among the more affluent societies than among primitive peoples (Mozden, 1965). In the United States cancer is the second leading cause of death, exceeded only by cardio-vascular diseases. Regarding the incidence of cancer, this statement from the American Cancer Society (1970) is sobering in the magnitude it suggests:

> More than 52 milion Americans now living will eventually have cancer: one in four persons according to the present rates. Cancer will strike over the years in approximately two of three famiiles. In the 70's there will be an estimated 3.5 million cancer deaths, 6.5 million new cancer cases, and 10.0 million under medical care for cancer (p. 3).

As the life span increases, the problem of cancer increases. The development of the means to prolong life coupled with the current trends to restrict births will tend to increase the proportion of the population most susceptible to the ravages of cancer.

Treatment Success

The picture of cancer is a grim one indeed. Each year thousands die or become disabled by it. However, the prospective rate of cure over time presents a more encouraging situation:

In the early 1900's few cancer patients had any hope of cure. In the late 1930's fewer than one in five was being saved—that is, alive five years after first being treated. Ten years later one in four was being saved. Since 1956, the ratio has been one in three. The gain from one to four to one to three currently amounts to some 54,000 lives each year. Of every six persons who get cancer today, two will be saved and four will die. Numbers 1 and 2 will be saved. Number 3 will die but might have been saved had proper treatment been received in time. Numbers 4, 5, and 6 will die of cancers which cannot yet be controlled; only the results of research can save these patients. This means that about half of those who get cancer could and should be saved—by early diagnosis and prompt treatment. Thus, the immediate goal of cancer control in the country is the annual saving of 325,000 lives, or half of those who develop cancer each year (American Cancer Society, 1970, p. 4).

However, it should be noted that this same publication points out that there are 1,500,000 Americans alive today, who have been cured of cancer. An additional 700,000 cancer patients diagnosed and treated within the past five years will live to be counted as cured. This means that there are more than 2,000,000 Americans cured of cancer.

While many people will survive their attacks of cancer, the treatment may have caused a loss of limb or radical alteration of some body function that requires major rehabilitative adjustments. Rehabilitation must develop and refine such techniques, skills, and facilities as will keep pace with the needs of this problem.

INDICATIONS FOR REHABILITATIVE INVOLVEMENT

The problems presented by cancer are no doubt manifold and to an extent overlapping. The presenting physiologic symptoms, of course, command the initial attention of the patient and those involved in his treatment. Usually these physiologic abnormalities were the impetus in causing the patient to seek medical advice and in such cases usually the fear of cancer is a very strong component. As the disease progresses the physical problems become more apparent and are more debilitating, painful and worrisome. Regardless of his knowledge or sophistication, the person experiencing the physiologic effects of cancer knows he has something seriously wrong with him. He may know, suspect, or even deny that he has cancer but the deep concern is always present. Those in whom cancer has been diagnosed by various means at the time may have minimal or no symptoms. Upon learning of their diagnosis, they in a sense join those in whom the ravages of the disease are more apparent in that they must come to grips with their new situation.

How the patient responds to this situation is, indeed, critical. No doubt, a basic question concerns the extent to which the subject is aware of his condition. Does he know he has cancer and does he know the extent of his involvement with it? What is his attitude toward cancer? If it is one of fear he may hesitate to seek aid until the chance of optimum care is past. Or, even after seeking aid his fears may dominate his thoughts and behavior to the point of rendering him ineffectual.

If his attitude toward cancer is one of revulsion, he may devalue himself and withdraw from all possible social inter-action. The attitude of self-pity is likewise present. "Why did this happen to me?" is a common question reflecting this point of view. In addition to these fears and attitudes the cancer patient is often confronted with the loss of a body part, change in function and appearance, and marked limitation of previously enjoyable and satisfying activities. Such a person has indeed suffered a loss and his reaction to this loss is a definite factor in his overall adjustment.

The person who suffers a loss of a body part, loss of or impairment of a function, or disfigurement not only suffers the inconvenience of not being able to do what he could do formerly, but he suffers a psychological loss as well. As others without these limitations may look upon the injured with pity and accord-ingly devalue them, so the person afflicted may come to pity and devalue himself. If he feels that he is repulsive to others he will likely become repulsive to himself, and this may interfere with what would be normal social relations (Demke, 1952).

It is possible that people who have sustained such a loss never get to the point where they can fully accept it. It does seem important to recognize that such a person may equate his personal loss with his personal worth. It is imperative that these two be kept separate so that even in the face of substantial loss the individual can still regard himself as a valuable member of society.

The main problem appears to be that the noninjured is considered to be the norm or model toward which all should orient themselves. Modern advertising stresses the perfection, beauty, and strength of the young and whole with the implication that we should all be like that. Most of us are not. Nonetheless, there is a tendency to view these near-perfect states as the ideal toward which we should all strive. The feelings one has about himself are crucial and, consequently, are the concern of physician and counselor alike.

The above comments tend to reflect the negative aspects of a subject's attitude. There is also the positive side in which the individual knows his condition, is accepting whatever treatment is appropriate, and is trying to get on with his life in the best way he can. The point is, the attitude of the subject is an important fact to be considered in both treatment and rehabilitation.

Another problem area presented by cancer concerns the counselor himself. What is the extent of his familiarity with cancer, the extent of his information, and the nature and magnitude of the problems they represent to the particular subject? What are the counselor's attitudes toward cancer? Since he is typically not a medical person, his attitudes—fears, biases, values, and so forth—may roughly parallel those of the client. If the counselor sees the problem as offering little or no hope for a lifetime that would merit substantial rehabilitative effort, there may be a disinclination on the part of the counselor to become really involved in the rehabilitative process. The counselor is prone to think in terms of longevity and function in relation to employment and his attitudes determine how he interprets this in regard to particular subjects.

From a rehabilitative point of view, the differences in cancer subjects is profound. There is no doubt small commonality among them and consequently there is no special counseling technique likely to serve them all. The differences in the disease itself as it affects the individual, coupled with the idiosyncratic reaction to it combine to make the rehabilitative problems very unique indeed. For subjects for whom a cure cannot be achieved, the pertinent medical and counseling questions would relate to what can be done to allay symptoms, prolong life and well being, and permit significant rehabilitation in terms of economic and family needs.

SHOULD THE PATIENT BE TOLD?

In working with cancer patients the question usually arises, "Should the patient be told that he has cancer?" There is no single right answer to this question, but there are a number of considerations that should be kept in mind when confronted with this problem. Cancer is a disease that is often thought by the public to be incurable and associated with untold agony, suffering, and death. Further, a knowledge of the diagnosis may only cause undue worry, depression, fear, and anxiety; and by withholding this information the patient may be spared considerable mental anguish and trauma.

Those actively working with cancer patients are well aware that this is not usually the case. There are many who have been cured of cancer and countless others who have had their lives significantly prolonged and have been able to function in an essentially normal manner. There is also the question of whether withholding the diagnosis actually does present or decrease the mental strain associated with the disease and whether there are other significant factors entering into the decision to follow this practice. Wangensteen (1950) has suggested that the family plays a big role in this decision in that, in addition to protecting the patient, they are actually protecting themselves from needless uneasiness. It is quite unlikely that withholding the diagnosis actually does cause the patient to be less concerned. The typical patient is reasonably sophisticated in his knowledge of certain aspects of medicine. Most people know the warning signs of cancer and when they have an illness which does not remit and have to undergo radical treatment they usually are very suspicious that they have cancer even though they might have been told otherwise.

Consideration must also be given to whether patients want to know and whether it is harmful for them not to know. An interesting survey of this question was carried out by Kelly and Friesen (1950). They surveyed two groups of patients: one group with known cancer and another group in whom there was no evidence of cancer. Of these subjects who did not have cancer, 82 percent said they would want to be told if it were to be diagnosed in them, and 14 percent said they would not want to be told. In the group with cancer, 89 percent said they would prefer to know about having cancer themselves. In regard to telling others with cancer, 73 percent of the cancer patients stated that they thought such people should be told; 4 percent said that people should not be told; and 20 percent thought that it could be individualized for each patient. Kelly and Friesen (1950) further state:

> Many of the patients remarked that they would be more willing and careful to follow directions in regard to necessary follow-up examinations if they knew they had cancer. Moreover, many of them stated that they worried more about the unknown and felt they preferred to know they had cancer, even if it was bad news, because it removed the indefiniteness of the situation (pp. 822-826).

Wright (1960) made an extensive study of the literature relating to this problem. After considering the available data, she offers these conclusions:

1. In by far the majority of cases, it is wiser to inform the patient of his condition than to conceal it.
2. Certainly where the patient is mature as a person, this course carries little risk.
3. Where the patient appears markedly immature and dependent, one may act more cautiously; but even in this case, if it is incumbent that the patient act realistically, sharing the state of affairs with him under the sustaining power of hope may be more efficacious.
4. Facing the situation realistically need not deny hope, for the two are psychologically not incompatible. Moreover, hope for a

possible favorable turn of events may even sustain one's resources in acting realistically in terms of the *probable* turn of events.

5. Further research is needed to enable the practitioner more reliably to select those cases where concealment is desirable. We ought not rest content with speculation, for this is an area amenable to investigation. Concealing difficult facts from children, for example, may or may not have the consequences we assume. (Our prejudice, probably shared by most people, is that children should be shielded, but let us remember that this is a prejudice until put to more objective test.)

6. As in all matters of counselor-client relationships, the effects of different rules of behavior or procedure depend on the attributes of the counselor as well as of the client. If the counselor has an abhorrence toward cancer, multiple sclerosis, or death, forces in him will resist mention of these facts. Or if the counselor devaluates the person who is ill or who has a disability, he will tend to overestimate the vulnerability of the patient to distressing information (pp. 360-361).

Family Aspects of Cancer

The cancer patient who lives in a family is surrounded— literally immersed—in a complex of attitudes related to cancer. It cannot be assumed that the family knows, understands and appreciates the fears of the cancer subject even though they are all living together in the same house. Further, it cannot be assumed that the family members will minimize their own anxieties over the fact that one of their members is so afflicted.

Indeed, the family members themselves may be very upset about the situation. They may have some fears about the possibility of becoming infected themselves since they are exposed in various ways to the disease. There may be a reluctance to touch the subject, his personal belongings, or even the dishes, towels, and other things he may use. There are also fears they may have about the hereditary aspects of the disease. If a family member has it, what are the prospects of other family members getting it, and what about the possibility of its being transmitted to any offspring? In addition, if the cancer problem has been in process any substantial amount of time there may be mounting medical bills that sorely drain the family resources.

These factors may produce fears, apprehension, and resentments on the part of the family toward the afflicted member. The subject is bound to sense these negative feelings on the part of the family members and this may be detrimental to his morale and to his response to the treatment process. This may produce a guarded relationship among the family rather than the supportive, loving relationship needed. Also, the client senses these family feelings and concerns. In his preoccupation with his own symptoms, particularly if the prognosis is guarded, he may feel that the family knows something he does not. This conclusion on his part may convince him that his condition is more serious than he thought.

So important is the family that if the client is not making the expected progress, the family situation may merit study. The generalization would be that all professional people concerned with a particular case must do all they can to help the family to accept the subject and to be prepared for his continued care.

Social and Community Aspects of Cancer

The cancer subject frequently demeans himself in various ways. He may be embarrassed by the nature of his affliction; and because of his own negative attitudes toward cancer, he may assume that everyone else feels the same way about it. This general feeling may cause him to avoid contacts with other people, particularly in such public gatherings as dances, games, meetings, theatres, etc. This may be especially true in instances where the individual has had a colostomy, wears an artificial bladder or other device, and fears an accident or worries about an odor that he may not be able to detect.

It seems that the basic problem relates to how the subject himself feels about cancer. The person who feels himself to be unworthy, distasteful to others, and so on, will tend to project these attitudes upon others and will behave accordingly. It is of crucial importance in his social adjustment to help the subject learn that many people so afflicted lead normal lives socially. Also, he can be taught the requisites of self-care that will minimize the possibility of having embarrassing situations develop.

Cancer is no longer considered to be solely a problem for the individual and his family. It is also a concern of society in general. It is important for the subject, his family, and all others involved in his care to be aware of the various resources in the community that may be of great practical value to him. The American Cancer Society and the various community health agencies are key sources of information about facilities and groups that might be of help in particular instances.

By the very nature of the disease, follow-up over a long period of time is of the utmost importance. This involves not only the motivation on the part of the subject to participate in the follow-up but also community facilities that would encourage this and in many instances make it possible.

RELATIONSHIP BETWEEN COUNSELOR AND PHYSICIAN

The counselor and the physician are inevitably tied closely together in working with the cancer patient. Each has a part to contribute and the other must not stand in the way.

The disease process itself involves medical questions that are basically within the province of the physician and should be left to him. Questions the physician should be permitted to respond to are these:

1. What is the nature of the disease itself? Explanations to the uninformed subject must, of course, be related to the depth and breadth of understanding of which the subject is capable at the moment.
2. What is the stage of the disease? Where is the disease so far as the particular patient is concerned?
3. What is the general outlook or prognosis? While the physician knows the general course to be expected, this has to be interpreted in terms of the particular patient.
4. Will treatment contemplated for the present or future require hospitalization or proximity to a treatment center?

5. How does the patient feel about his condition? Is he accepting it? Denying it? Resenting it? The question is whether the patient's attitude is conducive to the acceptance of treatment procedures.

Considerations more within the province of the counselor that would be useful in helping a particular client would include such information as the following:

1. aptitudes and interests of the subject
2. training facilities
3. employment opportunities
4. employment requirements
5. community agencies available to help the client
6. organizations oriented toward particular handicaps
7. the rehabilitation potential of a particular client

RELATIONSHIP BETWEEN COUNSELOR AND CLIENT

What the counselor does is more likely to convey his feelings about the patient than anything he might say. It isn't likely that the counselor could for very long deceive a client about how he sees the situation. The following considerations adapted from Lofquist (1957) may be of help to the counselor as he tries to work with the cancer client.

Does the counselor believe that his efforts will lead to the rehabilitation of the client? The counselor's actions will likely speak louder than his words. If the counselor is to appear sincere to the client, counseling must be complete and he must be consistent in his relationship with the client. If the counselor does not believe in the client's prospects, the client will likely know it.

If the counseling goal is a vocational one, the placement goals should be achievable as soon as practicable. Training programs should be arranged with this in mind. For practical reasons this will usually be compatible with the client's wishes because of lack of money and the uncertainty of the number of years he has available.

It is important that the plans for training and placement

take into consideration any existing physical limitations that the disease has imposed as well as any additional limitations that might develop.

It would seem to be important for the counselor to know how completely the family has been informed of the client's status since in counseling it is sometimes desirable to see the spouse and other family members.

The counselor should try to become as involved in the counseling process with the cancer client as he is with other clients. He must try to avoid letting his own fears about cancer become confused with those of the client.

At times, such a client may become quite aggressive. While such behavior may be quite disconcerting to the counselor, it must be considered that this behavior may be the client's way of expressing his fears. The counselor may take this as a signal that the personal feelings of the client need more or different attention. The counselor should not abandon the client in this moment of great need.

The counselor, of course, should be informed of the medical and surgical consequences of colostomy, facial disfigurement, plastic surgery, and so forth, and be prepared to help the client deal with the outcomes as he responds to them personally.

Many clients read extensively concerning their disability and may try to push the counselor into giving further information about the disease. It is not the place of the counselor to tell the client about the client's disease condition.

It scarcely needs to be said that the counselor should keep close liaison with the physician.

Conclusion

Since the report of the President's Commission on Heart Disease, Cancer and Stroke and the subsequent passage and enactment of the Heart Disease, Cancer and Stroke Amendment of 1965 significant emphasis has been given to the rehabilitation of cancer patients by the federal rehabilitative office. Miss Mary E. Switzer, then U. S. Commissioner of Vocational Rehabilitation, stated, "The rehabilitation of cancer patients has priority over almost anything else we are trying to do." She then pledged the resources of (RSA) to a redoubled effort to help victims of cancer back to productive and satisfying lives (*Rehabilitation Record,* 1966).

This reflects the general spirit and efforts of those concerned with cancer. Much has been done and much progress has been made but the problem has by no means been solved. Medical research is promising and we may be on the brink of discoveries that will provide medical solutions to the problem of cancer. In the meantime, we must work with what we know—early diagnosis and prompt treatment medically and an optimistic and constructive attitude psychologically and socially that will help the individual make the most of his life. Rehabilitation is a most significant vehicle in accomplishing this.

REFERENCES

Administrative Service Series 64-6, August 8, 1963.

American Cancer Society: *Teaching About Cancer.*

American Cancer Society: *Youth Looks At Cancer.*

Axtell, Lillian M.: Computing survival rates for chronic disease patients. *JAMA, 186*:1126, No. 13, December 28, 1963.

American Cancer Society: *Cancer Facts and Figures.* 1970.

Commissioner's Letter 68-5. August 29, 1967.

Commissioner's Letter 68-11. November 9, 1967.

Cutler, Sidney J. and Heise, Herman W.: Long-term end results of treatment of cancer. *JAMA, 216*:293, No. 2, April 12, 1971.

Demke *et al.,* Acceptance of Loss—Amputations. In Garrett, James F. (Ed.): *Psychological Aspects of Physical Disability. Rehabilitation Service Series Number 210.* Washington, D.C., Federal Security Agency, Office of Vocational Rehabilitation, U.S. Government Printing Office, pp. 80-86.

Gay, Richard L.: The Relationship Between Psychopathology and Cancer. *Dissertation Abstracts International* (Michigan State University), *21*: 4992 (8-8), February 1971.

Healey, J. E., Jr.: Changing philosophy toward rehabilitation. *Cancer Bull, 20*:2-3, January-February, 1968.

Henke, Walter: Evidence for viruses in acute leukemia and Burkitt's Tumor. *Cancer,* vol. 21, no. 4, April 1968.

Holleb, A. I.: Using the cancer cures we have now. *Today's Health,* April 1970.

Kelly, William D. and Friesen, Staley R.: Do cancer patients want to be told? *Surgery, 27*:822-826, no. 6, June 1950.

Knudson, Alfred G., Jr.: Genetics and cancer. *Postgrad Med,* vol. 48, no 5, November 1970.

Li, Frederck P. *et al.*: Familial ovarian carcinoma. *JAMA,* vol. 214, no. 8, November 23, 1970.

Lofquist, Lloyd H.: *Vocational Counseling with the Physically Handicapped.* New York, Appleton, 1957.

Mayer, Jean: Nutrition and cancer, part I. *Postgrad Med,* vol. 50, no. 4, October 1971.

Mayer, Jean: Nutrition and cancer, part 2. *Postgrad Med,* vol. 50, no. 5, November 1971.

Milt, Harry: Viruses and cancer. *A Cancer Journal for Clinicians,* vol. 19, no. 4, July-August 1969.

Mozden, Peter J.: Neoplasms. In Myers, Julian S. (Ed.): *An Orientation to Chronic Disease and Disability.* New York, Macmillan, 1965, p. 323.

Rehabilitation Record, vol. 7, no. 1, January-February 1966.

Research Brief of Significant Findings—Rehabilitation of Cancer Patients. New York, Memorial Hospital for Cancer and Allied Diseases.

Rusk, H. A.: Preventive medicine, curative medicine—the rehabilitation. *New Physician, 13*:165-167, 1964.

Shimkin, Michael B.: Duration of life on untreated cancer. *Cancer, 4*:1, 1951.

Wangensteen, Owen H. (Ed.): Should patients be told they have cancer. *Surgery, 27*:944-947, no. 6, June 1950.

Wright, Beatrice A.: *Physical Disability—A Psychological Approach.* New York, Harper and Brothers Publishers, 1960.

Chapter 2

MEDICAL AND PSYCHOLOGICAL

PROBLEMS IN THE REHABILITATION

OF THE CANCER PATIENT*

A. BEATRIX COBB

INTRODUCTION

CANCER IS PERHAPS the most baffling and challenging disability now referred for rehabilitation. It is baffling on two counts: medical and vocational.

On the medical side, cancer is surrounded by many unknowns. Despite recent dramatic advances in treatment and research, the cause of cancer is not clearly understood; the course of the disease varies extremely from organ to organ and from

---

* Special appreciation is here expressed to Malcolm J. Thomas, Jr., M.D. for invaluable assistance in the medical approach to cancer.

individual to individual; and the prognosis, although always guarded, now carries a hope for longer and longer, but uncertain, survival time.

The vocational frustration arises from two diverse sources. First, even when physical restoration seems successful, the nature of the disease still leaves the client and the rehabilitative counselor living under the very real threat of recurrence. Even if the individual seems physically able to cope with a previous or a new job, the question is always present, "For how long?"

The second vocational placement dilemma appears when the prospective employer is approached. If obvious physical mutilation or limitation due to the disease or treatment is present, it can pose a problem. Many are loath to accept an individual whose appearance may detract from business, or whose work may be interrupted by recurring illness.

As the survival time of the cancer patient has increased in more recent years, thought and effort have been turned to the quality of that survival (American Cancer Society, 1968). No longer is it sufficient to point with pride to the fact that more and more cancer patients are alive five or ten years after initial treatment of the disease. The question now arises: How are they alive? Are they invalids depending on others for emotional care and physical comfort? Are they living the life of a recluse, hiding from family and friends? Is the disease still under control? Have they picked up the prediagnostic threads of their lives and returned to gainful employment and rich personal existence?

No longer are physicians content to save a life; now they ask, "What kind of life?" In May of 1968, a national award-winning program, "Quality of Survival of the Cancer Patient," was held in Hartford, Connecticut. This conference was cosponsored by the Connecticut Division, Inc., American Cancer Society; the American Society of Surgeons; the Connecticut Society for Crippled Children and Adults; and the Vocational Rehabilitation Branch, United States Department of Health, Education and Welfare. At that conference, Dr. Charles Rogers, Memorial Hospital, New York City, epitomized the past and pointed to the future in these words:

I am saying that in our zealous endeavor to make more people survive longer, we have to a degree lost sight of a very necessary part of survival, and that is quality.

I offer you a quotation from the Bible . . . Matthew 16, verse 26: "For what does it profit a man if he gain the whole world, but suffer the loss of his soul " In the case of the cancer victim, I say to you: And what do we gain if we save a larger number, only to have them lead a life which for them is living hell (Kuehn, 1969, p. 17).

The *quality* of survival—is that not what rehabilitation is all about? The return of the disabled to meaningful personal and vocational self-sufficiency is the rehabilitative goal in any disability.

What is meant by "quality of survival?" In the above-mentioned conference, five pertinent factors were enumerated as essential to a quality survival (Kuehn, 1969, p. 1). These five included health, functions, comfort, emotional response, and economics.

The quality of the survivor's *health* encompassed not only recovery from onslaught and treatment of the disease, but also the general physical condition of the client five to ten years later. Is he up and around, with energy to live abundantly and to pursue gainful employment? Or, is he bedfast or without energy and motivation?

The topic of *functions* included the ability of the patient, in the follow-up period, to carry on with personal living chores and work assignments. Has he resumed prediagnostic work responsibilities, or is he limited in performance?

Comfort involves freedom from pain or the distress of limited activity. The quality of survival cannot be high if the patient endures debilitating pain or if he is constantly hampered in movement.

An often overlooked factor in the quality of success is that of *emotional response*. If the ravages of the disease or treatment have left the individual disfigured, his emotional reaction may interfere with his acceptance of the altered self. Included in this area are such items as his successful adjustment back into family and community living as opposed to becoming a recluse. Here, too, we must come to grips with the presence or absence of undue anxieties and fears centered around his future.

Finally, the *economic element* in the quality of survival is a pressing one. Even the initial expense of diagnosis and treatment is phenomenal. When there is added to this sum the cost of follow-up observations and treatment, plus the loss of income due to necessary absences to accomplish this treatment, the financial drain is considerable. If survival has meant bankruptcy for his family, the patient is not likely to look upon that survival as a "quality" one.

So, the role of rehabilitation in ensuring a quality survival in cancer is indeed a challenging one. Once the initial treatment is concluded and the patient is able to think in terms of picking up the joys and responsibilities of his life, rehabilitation can add much to the qualty of that living. A return to the world of work brings emotional relief and financial assistance. It allows the patient to focus on overcoming physical limitations and psychological anxieties in the process of preparing for return to gainful employment. The pain becomes more bearable; the limitations become more acceptable; the health status improves; and the emotional fears lessen as he once again assumes even partial financial responsibility for himself and for those he loves.

Little is known, however, about the ways and means to ensure this quality of survival. In many instances, the patient can return to his old job when he is physically and emotionally ready. In some cases, although he is physically and psychologically capable, the employer and his co-workers are not ready to accept him. In other cases, new jobs with preplacement training are indicated. In a few circumstances sheltered work situations are needed.

More well-planned experience and much action and research are needed before this challenge can be adequately met. Agency and medical personnel alike are still in early exploratory stages of rehabilitation work with cancer patients. Communication between the two groups is still difficult, though in their own way, representatives of each are earnestly trying to work with the other. Agency personnel are understandably unfamiliar with the medical parameters involved in this complex disability. Medical members of the team too often are not aware of the availability of services or of legal procedures guiding the work of the agency. Before much progress toward an integrated effort to enhance the quality of survival of the cancer patient can be accomplished, some concerted effort must be made to establish a pool of common knowledge (medical and rehabilitative) and to then systematically-expand this information in both directions.

Toward that goal, this chapter will seek to bring together pertinent medical and psychological data which may assist the rehabilitative counselor, or the family member, in a better understanding of the physical and emotional problems the cancer patient must endure. Through this understanding it is hoped that communication between the counselor and the physician (or the family member) can improve, and that through this improved communication and insights, the quality of survival for the cancer patient will be enhanced in his home and his community.

DEFINITION OF CANCER

One of the many baffling factors surrounding cancer is the difficulty of defining the term precisely. Cancer is a collective term used to describe all malignant neoplasms arising in the body tissue (WHO, 1966). Since cancers differ widely when associated with diverse organs or structures of the body, it is not possible at present to formulate a specific cause of cancer. The Medical Dictionary (Dorland, 1951) defines cancer as "a cellular tumor the natural course of which is fatal and usually associated with formation of secondary tumors" (p. 223). The report of a World Health Organization Expert Committee (1966) defines cancer as a "protean disease" and further states that a proper understanding of its many manifestations is essential to good clinical management (p. 5).

Such definitions give little satisfaction to one experiencing cancer, or one seeking to help an individual who has the disease. So much mystery and dread, so many unknowns surround the term that it is understandable that the diagnosis strikes terror to the hearts of those stricken and those who love them.

Perhaps following a comparison that leads from known factors to less known ones could bring a clearer understanding of this disease to all concerned. It is accepted that the normal cell grows in connection with that part of the body in which it has specific function. For instance, as the body develops in the uterus of the mother, the cells that make up the arms, hands, etc., take food, multiply, and grow in harmony with other cells and organs until the arm, hand, or other members of the body are complete. Upon completion of the body member, and from that time forward, the cells continue to take food and multiply but also *die* according to a regular cycle. In this way the body member is maintained, but does not continue to grow to massive size.

Cancer cells, however, do not grow in harmony with the cells from which they are derived or with the organs in which they arise, but operate in a lawless, unorthodox manner. So instead of maintaining order and coordination among the body organs, the cancer cells continue to grow and multiply. They relentlessly invade the body structures, taking over the food supply by diverting the blood and lymph channels to supply themselves rather than allowing the normal delivery of oxygen and food to the essential organs of the body. Thus they damage the organs adjacent to, or containing, the new invading mass. The result is body weight loss, anemia, and decreased tissue function; so the savage cancerous horde sweeps over the weakened body much as a plundering army spreads over a conquered land.

Once the cancer cells have set up operations within the body, they spread through the blood-stream, the lymph channels, and locally to adjacent structures. Again like an invading army they divide, conquer and colonize. When the cancer cells are carried by blood-stream or lymph channels to parts of the body distance from the original site, the new colony of spread is referred to as "metastasis."

Under a microscope, this rebellious cancer cell resembles the normal cell but appears to be immature (not fully developed). It looks like embryonal cells. The younger the appearance of the cell, the more vicious seems its power of tissue invasion. This accounts for the fact that cancers differ in rate of spread. Some are said to be "fast-growing" and spread over the body rapidly. Others are termed "slow-growing" and may take years to overwhelm the body functioning.

Since the term *cancer* includes all malignant tumors, the usual practice is to speak of "different cancers affecting different organs or structures" (WHO, 1966, p. 5). Because this is true, cancer has been said to be not one disease, but many. The symptoms, course, treatment, and prognosis are related specifically to the organ invaded and its normal function. All of this seems to add up to a fatal condition surrounded by dangerous unknowns or little knowns. The picture is not as dark as these facts would seem to indicate. Indeed, "it has been estimated that one cancer in every three is of a type for which cure by the best existing method is feasible" (WHO, 1966, p. 5).

Perhaps further clarification of the meaning of the disease known as cancer will develop as the discussion continues to the complex procedures of medical diagnosis of the condition. The emotional impact of the diagnosis of cancer on the patient and his family will also be considered.

MEDICAL AND PSYCHOLOGICAL IMPLICATIONS IN THE DIAGNOSIS OF CANCER

In cancer perhaps more than any other disease, an early diagnosis is significant. Speaking of cancer, medical experts have coined a prophetic saying: "The first chance to cure is the best chance to cure" (WHO, 1966, p. 6). Far too often, and contributing considerably to the fatality of the disease, the diagnosis is not made until the malignancy is widespread. This fact is not usually due to inept medical service, but to the insidious nature of the disease itself. In many instances, the cancer has reached advanced stages before the patient becomes aware of a difficulty sufficient to take him for medical advice.

The Importance of Early and Accurate Diagnosis

The urgent need for early diagnosis is also centered in the complexity of the disease. Cancers not only differ in tissues of origin and structural appearances, but also arise from different causes, having varying clinical courses, and appearing in individuals of divergent age, of either sex, and of differing physiological and psychological characteristics. Proper treatment for the specific cancer can be initiated only when correct and comprehensive information is available to the treating physician.

Again, cancer is said to be not one disease, but many diseases, as determined by the organ (site) in which it originates. These diversified malignancies respond in specific ways to various treatments. Effective diagnosis, therefore, is concerned with the identification of a specific type of cancer (histological), affecting a certain organ (site) or structure, of a particular individual of a specific sex and age, with unique physiological and psychological characteristics. The extent of the onslaught of the malignancy, and the presence or absence of metastasis must also be known. All of these factors are of extreme importance in the diagnosis and prognosis (medical prediction of the course and termination of the disease). Only with this information can definitive treatment be initiated.

It is really obvious that this comprehensive evaluation can be done best in a well-equipped center where cancer-trained physicians and ancillary staff members are available. The fact is, however, that most cancers are first tentatively diagnosed by a family physician. The patient may not suspect the presence of cancerous material and the family physician uncovers the possibility in routine examinations or in exploratory procedures. Such a patient is referred *immediately* to a center or clinic where adequate equipment and medical specialists are available. The lives of many have been saved, or lengthened, by such prompt referrals.

One of the most treacherous traits of cancer is its ability to remain hidden until the functioning of a vital organ is interrupted. This gives the malignant growth opportunity to establish itself firmly in the primary site, and even set up colonies in adjacent organs or tissues (metastasis) before its presence is recognized. Often the symptoms mask the true condition by assuming physical signs peculiar to other diseases. For instance, cancer of the breast may appear as the cystic mass sometimes present in mammary tissues; or, cancer of the lung has at times been honestly diagnosed as tuberculosis. Cancer of the cervix often mimics menopausal indications, etc.

Lay people, puzzled by the intricate peculiarities of the

disease, sometimes ask, "What does a cancer look like?" Or, "Why do you need a biopsy (a surgically excised bit of tissue from the suspected site) before a diagnosis can be made?" If the reader will review the section on definition of cancer, the answer is obvious. It is *only* when the tissues can be studied under a microscope in order to determine the structure of the cells themselves that definitive diagnosis can be made. Even then, this study must be done by a highly trained, skillful pathologist, or errors may arise.

Psychological Impact of Diagnosis of Cancer

All of the intricate medical procedures mentioned above are being carried out on people. Even the most stoic individual dreads the discomfort and indignity of a thorough physical examination when it is a routine procedure. When the patient realizes that something serious is going on, anxiety looms and permeates his being.

Threat of the Intimate Meaning of the Diagnosis

When the diagnosis has been made as cancer, the patient is precipitated into a state of biological defenselessness that is almost intolerable. There is no simple physiologic explanation of cancer, and there can be no firm assurance of recovering. So the patient comes face to face with a threat that is consistent with his own intimate knowledge of the meaning of cancer.

Cancer means many things to many people (Cobb, 1959). In a study of forty patients with a known cancer diagnosis, there seemed to be a continuum of anxiety experienced, ranging from "no appreciable threat" through a vague nonspecific fear to a verbalized specific menace, and ending in what seemed to be an intelligent, controlled anxiety.

No appreciable threat at the diagnosis of cancer was reported by 12.5 percent of the sample Cobb studied. An evaluation of the reasons for no anxiety given by this group indicated that they were not informed about cancer. Several individuals simply were from uneducated families where their life-styles precluded their having been reached by cancer education literature. They said such things as: "I thought it was just one of them little old tumors," or "I didn't see how it could be serious; it didn't hurt me none." A few well-educated members of the group were lulled into a false security by such specific medical names as "melanoma" and "Hodgkin's Disease" and did not at first connect these names with malignancies.

Approximately 25 percent of the population investigated reported vague nonspecific fears focused around the diagnosis of cancer. When their reports were analyzed, it was obvious that for the most part this fourth of the group really went into shock when the diagnosis was revealed to them. There seemed to be a lack of anxiety that was really an inability to verbalize fears. Several said such things as: "It just seemed like one of those things that you think can't happen to you," or "I had mixed emotions about it." Others simply repeated, "I was scared to death." One gave a vivid description of acute shock (Cobb, 1959):

> I guess I was just petrified when he (the doctor) told me. I came through the operation in a stage of what seemed like exaltation, or joy, and felt completely unafraid. I seemed at peace with the world, but didn't seem attached to it. I made up poetry all the time, and fell back on religion. I was living in a world above earthy woes. . . . Then, it wore off and I came back to earth with a bang. Now, I realize that I was simply in a daze. I was so petrified, I didn't know what was happening to me really (Cobb, 1959, p. 276).

More than half (52.5 percent) of the sample reported a specific, personal threat. This specific menace was *death*. To then cancer was synonymous with death. One man expressed the consensus: "If you get it, it ain't no use to run to a doctor, for he can't do nothing for you anyway. . . . You're gonna die. I seen my old daddy die of the same thing, just like I go. . . . I know (Cobb, 1959, p. 277).

Another younger man described the feeling he had by saying, "It was just like walking up to a sleeping man, shaking his hand and saying to him, 'You're gonna die right now!'" One spinster in her late fifties was precipitated into a psychotic episode by the diagnosis. She said, "I want to go home. I no can get well. I have chickens and a cow at my house. I have flowers. . . .

They are so pretty (voice breaks, tears threaten, and then she sits up suddenly rigid and claws violently at the lump in her throat—thyroid cancer). I have cancer. I have cancer here. I die. I know, I die" (Cobb, 1959, p. 278).

The patient was hospitalized in a mental institution several days later. After treatment there, a successful operation was performed and the thyroid cancer excised.

To a small number in this specific category of threat, the menace was not so much death *per se* as it was punishment for prior sins. They said such things as, "I've been wicked all my life. I had it coming to me." Or, "It's a disgrace sent on me for my sins."

> One black woman was convinced that God had sent cancer of the breast upon her because she sold beer at her "eating place." She sent for a "prayer cloth" through the mail and waited nine weary and painful months, while the tumor in her breast fulminated and broke into a running sore, hoping that God would forgive and heal her (Cobb, 1959, p. 278).

Only 10 percent of the group studied accepted the diagnosis of cancer with intelligent, controlled anxiety. Proper knowledge of the course of cancer and the medical advances toward its control seemed to determine this reaction. One man put it simply: "I know about malignancies. My wife had one. You face such things, get the best possible medical care, and keep it controlled" (Cobb, 1959, p. 278).

One patient expressed her reaction succinctly:

> I was absolutely petrified when this friend told me I had cancer, but I had the good sense to call my doctor, and after I had talked to him, I felt so much better. He was blunt, but he gave me courage and hope. He said you have met hard problems before and this is just another one. You are an adult, and I know you would want to know. I want you to put your house in order before you go . . . for treatment. . . . I mean your spiritual house as well as your mental and physical house, and then go . . . and give those doctors everything you have in you to help them get you well. You know the doctor can do only so much and then it's up to you. I appreciated that so much in the days to come. I talked with other doctors; I read; and I found out what my chances were, what they had to

offer in the way of treatment; and then I set myself to help the doctors help me (Cobb, 1959, p. 279).

To be told you have cancer, then, may mean different things. The counselor or family member must know the specific fear the patient visualizes if he is to give maximum emotional support. Often, the anxiety experienced is realistic; in some instances, it is based upon misinformation which can be corrected. As has been reported, a picture of no appreciable threat may be based upon ignorance of the course and prognosis of the disease. What seems to be stolid acceptance or cheerfulness may be shock that defies verbalization. Often some of this discomfort can be relieved by talking about realistic risks of the disease and what can be done for the patient. The focus of the debilitating anxiety may be death, *per se* or guilt over past sins. If so, correct information and exposure of the fancied fears to the light of scientific advances and hope may push this individual over into the desired category of controlled fear of the disease. A controlled, intelligent fear is to be desired. It assists the patient in resisting the onslaught of the disease by intelligent cooperation with the physician in the treatment schedule. It also assists in alleviating debilitating anxiety and converting it into a mobilizing energy which may be used to combat the disease.

Psychologic Meaning of the Organ Involved

The emotional significance of the organ involved (which may be destroyed by the disease or treatment) adds to the impact of the diagnosis. This trauma is especially debilitating when the organ or structure has symbolic impact. A woman faced with the loss of a breast feels that her sexual attractiveness is threatened. Often a young woman feels she is losing the right to love and marriage with the loss of a breast. She cannot countenance the possibility of the look of admiration turning to repulsion in the eyes of the man she loves.

Married women often fear they will lose their husbands as a result of the body mutilation. In fact, a number of divorces, and separations, have occurred for this reason. It is plausible, however, that the break in the marriage relationship was as much due to the attitude and fear of the wife, as to the change or repulsion in the husband. With proper talking and feeling through the projected loss and clarification of the symbolic meaning of the organ, the marriage might have been saved. On numerous occasions, when the husband and wife were led to discuss the problem candidly with the guidance of the counselor, the marriage relationship was actually reinforced. One brave young man, whose initial reaction was one of horror and distaste (because the scar offended his esthetic sense) came to the counselor, worked through his emotions, and arrived at his own basic decision that love was stronger than any disfigurement. With his support and the knowledge of the depth of his love, the wife made a remarkable recovery. They weathered the threat and left the hospital more secure in their relationship than ever before.

Cancer of the cervix carries a deep symbolic significance also. Cobb (1959) reported a case wherein the patient felt the radical surgery essential to control of the cancer was a violation of her womanhood. She told of a poignantly sad episode of the last night before her operation. Feeling that this was to be her last night as a whole woman, she wore her wedding gown (she had only been married a short six months). Her husband, she said, scoffed at her, but "that is the way I felt. You go in there, knowing that when you come out you can no longer function as a normal woman. It's like taking away your womanhood" (Cobb, 1959, p. 280).

When the husband places great value on a large family, cancer of the cervix carries an added threat to the patient. Often a woman needs reassurance that normal physical, marital relationships are possible following treatment.

Emotional reactions related to the symbolic meaning of the organ invaded are not limited to women. Men see cancer of the prostate and of the genitalia as a menace to their manhood as well. The loss of sexual potency is often even more traumatic to a man than to a woman.

The counselor, family members, and the medical team all could profit from knowledge of the possible emotional impact of the diagnosis of cancer to the patient. This information should include the intimate meaning of the word "cancer" to the patient, as well as the symbolic significance of the organ or structure involved. Medical management may be facilitated by this knowledge and much of the emotional trauma of the patient ameliorated. As the physician, the counselor, and the family members listen to the patient and respond to his verbalized and unspoken fears, the way is paved for acceptance of the diagnosis and intelligent participation of the patient in treament.

TREATMENT OF MALIGNANT TUMORS

Treatment of cancer is complex and varied. As has been stated, often the treatment itself is a frightening experience for the patient. This phase of the management of patients with a malignant disease will be approached from two directions. First, the complicated choices of techniques for medical treatment will be presented. Second, the emotional impact, on the patient, of experiencing the treatment, will be explored.

Medical Treatment of Cancer

Once the diagnosis is made, the preparation of an individual plan for management of the disease becomes the first and most important step in treatment. The extent and form of treatment should be devised in light of the specific circumstances of the patient and in his best interest. The plan must be flexible to the point that modifications may be made in an expedient manner to cope with any emergency that might arise.

So complex is cancer that it is prudent that the plan be devised and treatment be carried out by a team of specialists. This team should include a surgeon, a radiotherapist, an internist (or family physician), a pathologist, a psychologist or psychiatrist, and a rehabilitative counselor.

The emotional response of the patient to the disease must be given careful attention by a physician (or a psychiatrist or psychologist if the reaction is severe) in order to enlist the confidence and cooperation of the patient and his family in the treatment plan. The effect the disease and/or the treatment will, or may, have on the career of the patient should be frankly discussed, and the rehabilitative counselor should be brought into the team prior to initial treatment, if feasible. This gives the patient a hope for a return to normal wage earning upon recovery which can add to motivation to overcome the disease and decrease the degree of depression during the critical days following radical surgery or extensive radiotherapy.

Again, prior to initiation of treatment, the team needs to review the precise clinical extent of the disease, the anatomical site of the original tumor, and the presence or absence of distant spread (metastasis) of the disease. In deep-seated cancers (i.e. cancer of the stomach, lungs, breast, etc.) specific assessment can be made only through surgical exploration and pathological examination of the tissues involved.

The pathologist, then, is a most essential member of the treatment team. Pathological examination of the cells makes possible a definitive diagnosis of cancer. Through pathological examination the type of cancer is determined. It should be pointed out that although cytological and clinical examinations may *indicate* the presence of cancer, the diagnosis cannot be *confirmed* until the histopathological examination has been completed and the structure of the tumor clarified.

For instance, when cancer of the breast is suspected, immediate histological examination of sections obtained by limited resection is accomplished. While the patient is still on the operating table, the report of the pathological findings (benign or malignant) determines whether or not radical mastectomy is to be done.

In all instances, the pathologist should examine the entire specimen removed during surgery. This examination gives the treatment team essential information as to the histological characteristics of the tumor, the type of reaction in the surrounding tissues, the extent of the cancerous growth to surrounding structures, and the adequacy of the excision.

A full microscopic examination should also be made of any lymph nodes removed in order to determine whether or not there is metastatic spread of the disease. This evidence may determine whether or not radiotherapy and/or chemotherapy should follow the surgery.

The treatment plan should also take into consideration several biological characteristics of the client. The physical fitness and the age of the patient must be considered. Again, in cancer of the breast, such conditions as pregnancy and lactation demand extreme caution in treatment since some tumors seem to evidence extremely rapid growth at that time.

Taking into consideration all of these factors, a team decision as to the preferred treatment is made. The patient then becomes the major responsibility of the specialists (surgeon, if surgery is decided upon; radiotherapist, if radiation is chosen; or the internist or endocrinologist, if chemotherapy is indicated). Stehlin and Beach (1966), a surgeon and a psychiatrist, respectively, writing on the topic "Psychological Aspects of Cancer Therapy" spoke of the plan in terms of the emotional needs of the patient: "A reasonable plan is one in which optimism and hope for cure are combined with reality. Too little optimism is more reprehensible than too much" (p. 101).

TYPES OF TREATMENT

Five types of treatment may be utilized in the battle to save the life of an individual diagnosed to have cancer. Usually, the treatment of choice is surgery. Radiotherapy is used extensively in combating cancer, sometimes as the initial treatment, and often as supplementary to surgery. Recently, chemotherapy, although not considered able to produce a permanent cure, has been found to have considerable application in cancer treatment (WHO, 1966, p. 22). Also quite recently hormone therapy (particularly in instances of cancers of the breast, cervix and prostate) has been utilized successfully in the control of cancer. The fifth form of treatment is known as combined therapy. Combinations of surgery, radiotherapy, chemotherapy and even hormone therapy have been used in the overall management of the patient through the course of the disease. Each of these forms of treatment will be briefly discussed.

Surgery

Because of the vicious nature of the disease, surgery is the preferred treatment (WHO, 1966). This is particularly true if the patient presents himself for medical care early in the history of his disease, while the cancer is still encapsulated in the primary site (no metastasis to distant parts of the body). Three types of surgery are performed in cancer: diagnostic, curative, and palliative. The nature of each will be reviewed.

Diagnostic Surgery

Diagnostic surgery is performed in order to establish a correct diagnosis. This procedure may be a simple biopsy or an exploratory operation.

A biopsy involves the incision and removal of tissue from a lesion (tumor) for pathological examination. As previously mentioned, the pathological examination of the biopsied material helps to establish a correct diagnosis and gives essential facts which may determine the nature and extent of treatment needed.

When all medical investigations fail to establish a definitive diagnosis when malignancy is suspected or must be ruled out, surgery is sometimes recommended.

Curative Surgery

It was the consensus of the members of the expert committee of the World Health Organization (1966) that "the value of surgery in the treatment of cancer lies in the fact that in the great majority of cases the neoplasm is unicentric in origin. This being so, there is every prospect of cure if the tumor can be extirpated before it has metastasized" (p. 13).

Palliative Surgery

The purpose of palliative action is to relieve pain and discomfort or to prolong life. This type of surgery is carried out to help the patient, but it is not expected to cure. Surgical procedures are employed to resect infected, foul, bleeding or obstructive cancer tissues. Severance of sensory-nerve tracts, or alcohol nerve blocks are used to relieve intractable pain. Bypass operations in cancer-infiltrated gastrointestinal and urinary tracts are utilized to relieve obstructions. Palliative surgery may also be employed to enhance the degree of freedom from distress experienced by the patient found to be inoperable for cure upon exploratory operation. It has been shown that the removal of a primary tumor, in some cases, will cause regression of distant metastasis, relieving the patient of symptoms and complications and prolonging life.

In case of bone sarcoma, or soft-tissue malignancies, an amputation of an extremity may be considered a palliative operation. It should be pointed out, however, that a palliative resection can be useful only when the general condition of the patient is fairly good, and when the goal is to prolong life. If no sign of dissemination is present, procedures not palliative but curative may be carried out.

Radiotherapy

It has been estimated that radioatherapy is indicated in the management of at least 50 percent of all cancer patients (WHO, 1966):

> Radiotherapy depends for its action on the biological response if ionizing radiation. The immediate effect of ionizing radiation on tissue is a specific kind of physically induced inflammation, the degree of the reaction depending on the dosage of radiation to which the tissue has been exposed (p. 18).

The radiation works to damage the cancer, not through a cauterizing effect, but by selective damage of the malignant cells. Cancerous tumors are classified as radiosensitive, radioresistant, and intermediate. Radiosensitivity implies rapid regression in response to radiography. Radioresistant tumors are those that evidence limited or no regression when irradiated.

Radiotherapy, like surgery, is used as a palliative procedure as well as a curative process. When a cure is considered feasible according to the size of the tumor, every effort is expended to that end. Radiotherapy may be used before surgery to reduce the tumor to operable size. Surgery is then carried out to remove the primary site. Radiotherapy may also be utilized following surgery as a precaution against scattered malignant cells that might remain.

If the patient is considered incurable, relief from pain, ulceration, and so on, may be secured through irradiation. It may also be used in conjunction with drugs in such cases.

Chemotherapy

Treatment of cancer by drugs alone is not indicated when there is hope the tumor can be cured by surgery or irradiation. However, around 50 percent of malignant diseases are known to respond to chemotherapy, either used alone, or in combination with other forms of treatment. In the lymphomas, Hodgkin's Disease and the retinoblastomas, chemotherapy is often used in combination with other treatment when the disease is limited in extent. In the treatment of acute and chronic leukemia and multiple myeloma, chemotherapy may be used (WHO, 1966). When cancer is advanced and generalized, and other treatment cannot be accomplished, chemotherapy is widely used.

Intrapleural and intraperiotoneal chemotherapy have been utilized successfully for patients with pleural or ascitic effusions resulting from cancer. The fluid is drawn and the drug is introduced into the pleural or peritoneal cavity. This procedure often reduces the rapidity of the recurrence.

Regional chemotherapy (extracorporeal circulation to perfuse the organ attacked with the chemotherapeutic agent) has been used in treatment of intractable cancer. This method is complicated.

Intra-arterial infusion in localized areas appears to have more promise in certain cancers. Both of these prodecures need further research (WHO, 1966).

Hormone Therapy

The first physiological substances known to influence the course of cancer are hormones. Hormone therapy is used both as additive and as suppressive treatment. Over the past twenty years, sex hormones have been used as additive treatment in cancer of the breast in females and prostate in males. Progesterone has been used in endometrial cancer and in acute and chronic leukemia. In malignant lymphoma, corticosteroids have proven of value.

Side effects of hormone administration represent a complication that requires medical consideration. Research to find a hormone free from these effects is under way. Investigations are also in progress attempting to identify hormone-dependency in types of cancer other than in the breast and prostate.

Combined Therapy

Many combinations of forms of treatment for cancer have been used through the years. Surgery plus radiotherapy, surgery plus chemotherapy, radiotherapy plus chemothreapy and other combinations have been tried.

Surgery Plus Radiotherapy

Surgery may be preceded or followed by radiotherapy or both may be performed. Preoperative radiotherapy may be used when the bulk of the tumor makes surgery difficult. The irradiation not only decreases the size of the malignancy, it reduces the risk of dissemination of cancer cells during the operation, by the obliteration of blood and lymphatic vessels surrounding the malignant site. Postoperative radiotherapy is based on the theory that isolated malignant cells may remain following operation, that can be killed more readily in isolation than in mass.

Breast cancer irradiation postoperatively is well established. Intra-uterine radiation before hysterectomy for adenocarcinoma of the *corpus uteri* is often used. Radon seeds and radioactive isotopes are widely used in combination with surgery.

Surgery Plus Chemotherapy

This combination seems advantageous in the management of some cancers (i.e. cancers of the ovary and breast). The drug may be given preceding, during, or following the operation. Chemotherapy is used in conjunction with surgery on the same premise that radiotherapy is utilized. First, it could be used to reduce the size of the tumor. Second, it could attack remaining cancer cells left in the body following operation. Much research should continue in this area.

Radiotherapy Plus Chemotherapy

The management of malignant lymphoma often requires the use of radiotherapy and chemotherapy combined. Radiotherapy is used as a curative treatment when the extent of the disease is limited. Chemotherapy assumes an important role when the cancer is widespread.

Surgery, Radiotherapy and Chemotherapy with Hormone Treatment

Inasmuch as breast cancer has been demonstrated to be hormone dependent, the use of hormone therapy has been added to the massive attack on this disease. Even more recently, knowledge relative to steroid excretion and the growth of breast cancer has also improved patient survival in cancer of the breast. Treatment for this disease, if it is widespread, then, may include surgery, radiotherapy, chemotherapy, and administration of hormones.

Team Treatment in Cancer

Treatment for cancer is a complex and challenging problem. The Expert Committee of WHO (1966) pointed out that cancer is definitely a team responsibility:

> The plan of treatment should be determined, not by a single specialist, but by a team, and the team approach should be adopted as widely as possible. The aim should be to employ, often in combination, techniques that wlil give the best results with the least upset to the patient. The team should have the necessary facilities for the proper diagnosis of cancer, including a well-equipped pathology laboratory capable of dealing with biopsies, urgent surgical biopsies, pathological examination of specimens taken at operation, and necropsies (p. 39).

PSYCHOLOGICAL IMPACT OF TREATMENT FOR CANCER

When the patient has accepted the diagnosis and agreed to recommended treatment, his emotional trauma is not ended. The very nature of the treatment poses the greatest threat of all. Radical surgery is usually advocated, and this sometimes means the loss of portions of the body that the patient has not associated with his problem. For instance, a patient with sarcoma may lose an entire leg, when to him the trouble seems localized on the ankle. A woman who has a small mass in her breast may awake from anesthesia to find that her breast has been removed. Intellectually, she knows this radical procedure was carried out to save her life, but an unreasonable emotional grief results.

Many patients are deathly afraid of surgery. Often this fear is based on the loss of consciousness under anesthesia and the horror of the knife cutting into their defenseless bodies. Sometimes it is realistic anxiety arising from having known someone who experienced the same procedure and being too keenly aware of what to expect.

Radiotherapy is also approached with uneasy anticipation. It is difficult for the lay person to understand how heavy dosages of irradiation can be delivered to the body without literally destroying it. The sound-proof rooms in which extensive irradiation is usually administered give an eery "feeling" to the treatment. Often the patient experiences nausea following irradiation. At times this nausea is a result of the physical impact of the therapy, but it may also be intensified or even a result of the emotional reaction to the unknowns of the radiotherapy.

Radioactive iodine seems an awesome mystery to most patients. They are asked to drink what appears to be a glass of strange-tasting water. Then they are warned of the presence of the radioactive substance in their bodies and may be isolated, or restricted as to visiting time. The next day, the geiger counter buzzes over them in an alarming manner. This is boring routine to the physicians and technicians, but it is dangerous magic to many patients.

Chemotherapy and hormone treatments precipitate psychological concerns. Anxiety-producing side effects of the drugs used heighten the psychological discomfort of the patient. Hormones and the cortisones bring about personality, as well as physical, changes that alarm the patient and his family.

Supportive Needs of the Patient During Treatment

During treatment, the cancer patient needs open communication lines between his physician, his family and himself. He needs to know *what* is going to be done, *how* it is going to be done, and *why*. If he has the answers to these urgent questions, he can relax and use his energy to meet the aftermath of the treatment.

Cobb (1962) reported a case where a young woman yanked the needle from her arm and refused to allow blood to be drawn for a laboratory test. She had not been told what was going on or why it was being done. An older man refused prostatic treatment because he did not understand how the procedure was to be accomplished. Much debilitating anxiety can be avoided by carefully maintained communication channels between the doctor, nurse and patient.

After surgery is over, the physician has a responsibility to discuss the results with the patient. Stehlin and Beach (1966) address themselves to this obligation:

> Intially, he (the patient) should be told merely "you came through the operation fine, and as soon as you feel more comfortable, we shall go over the whole matter. . . ." When the appropriate time arrives, the operative findings and procedures should be briefly and simply described.
>
> The surgeon should therefore be prepared for such questions as "Did you get it all?" "Had it spread?" "Will it come back?" and "What are my chances?" Again he (the doctor) must appreciate the patient's extreme anxiety and attempt to cope with it in an intelligent and realistic manner (p. 101).

Psychological Needs of the Incurable Cancer Patient

The course of incurable cancer is usually a series of remissions, during which time the patient feels much better, only to be followed by a recurrence which precipitates treatment again. The patient needs consistent emotional support to assist him toward an acceptance and enjoyment of the period of remission when he can live fairly normally, as well as an acceptance of the surety of recurrence, and relief that he has a medical haven to which he can return when that time comes. Many patients make remarkable adjustments to these cycles of health and illness. They seem to place the responsibility in the hands of the medical team, relax and enjoy the pain-free days, and with faith return for another miracle when the cycle turns against them.

Faith in the medical team and hope for a cure around the corner seem to be major ingredients that make for a cooperative attitude and good mental health in the patient. Stehlin and Beach (1966) state, "If the incurable patient is to gain the utmost benefit from the surgeon's care, their relationship must be a close one, and this is possible only in an atmosphere of mutually free and open communication" (p. 101). Speaking of hope, they continue:

> We surgeons who are constantly dealing with the physical aspects of cancer should realize that the words "incurable" and "hopeless" are not synonymous. To tell a patient that his condition is hopeless is both cruel and technically incorrect. Incurability is a state of the body, whereas hopelessness is a state of mind, a giving up—a situation that must be avoided at all cost. A patient can tolerate knowing he is incurable; he cannot tolerate hopelessness (p. 102).

One might well question the source of hope upon which the incurable patient may draw. Again Stehlin and Beach (1966) have a meaningful theory:

> The answer is simply that he can hope things will be better. The nature and the quality of his hope will be influenced by (1) the patient's attitude toward cancer, (2) the physical factors associated with his disease and the method available for treatment, (3) his attitude in general toward life and his will to life, and (4) the attitude and personality of the physician (p. 102).

There can always be hope for control of the disease, if cure is not feasible. Even when hope for control of the disease is no longer reasonable, there is still hope for comfort. These hopes may be met through medical management:

> by a change of narcotics, or the addition of a tranquilizer, an adjustment of electrolyte inbalance, measures to improve hydration and nutrition, transfusions, attention to malodorous ulcers, stabilization of fractures, physical therapy and, if feasible, efforts directed toward ambulation (Stehlin and Beach, 1966, p. 103).

It is within the parameters of the third quality of hope (attitude toward life and the will to live) that the contribution of the psychiatrist, the psychologist, clergyman, social worker and/or rehabilitative counselor is most pertinent. It is at this point that the patient and the team members must come to terms with the intimate meaning that death has for each of them. If the team member in the supportive role has not made a personal peace with the concept of death, he may be threatened and ill at ease with the patient. Cobb (1962) speaks of the dilemma in which the inexperienced psychologist finds himself at such times:

> Paradoxically, the most devastating and at the same time the most rewarding experience of working with cancer patients comes from the relationship leading to an acceptance of the inevitability of death. It is devastating because no sensitive person can work with the deep emotional problems of another human being in the process of preparing for death without reeling at times under the impact of stark separation trauma. It is rewarding because there is never a greater need for emotional support, for emphatic understanding, even for moments of diversion, than one finds in the patient getting ready for death. Between devastation and reward, it takes courage, tenacity, and humility to maintain a counseling relationship when the goal is acceptance and adjustment to the finality of death (pp. 151-152).

Too often the supportive team member (professional or family) hesitates because he doesn't know what to do or say. Three comforting rules-of-thumb may reassure him. First, the most important rule is to listen. Listen not only to the words but to the feelings made apparent by a tone of voice, a sad look, a tear. Many times the patient only needs a sympathetic ear to work through his own problems. These problems may have to do with his family. What will happen to them when he is gone haunts his waking hours.

Here a family member, or members, can give more comfort than anyone. It is, however, one of the most difficult things a person may ever do to talk quietly and with as little emotion as possible about closing the family circle when the patient is gone. One farmer worked out a dated diary during this period, in which he went through a year, writing in the dates that cotton should be planted, the hogs sold, the wheat planted and harvested, the insurance and taxes paid, etc. When he had finished it, he went through it carefully first with his wife, then with their two teenage children. He gained relief from the planning and discussion and the family lived by it for a number of years.

Putting one's house in order financially and spiritually are urgent problems to many. The helper can assist by contacting individuals who can help, such as a lawyer for financial planning, or a clergyman for spiritual comfort. This is done only if the patient wishes it to be done, but settling these affairs often brings a peace of mind that eases the confrontation with death.

Second, the individual in the nurturing role may give information that concerns the patient. For instance, the patient may want to know how much longer the treatment he is enduring will continue, and if something else will be done when it is discontinued. Through close contact with the physician, these questions can be answered. The patient may wish to see a child or a friend but wonders if a visitor could or should come. He may just need to be reassured that the medical team is not going to give up, and that, as Stehlin and Beach (1966) have said, even beyond hope for control there is hope for comfort. *Always* there is the consideration and dignity to which he is entitled as an important human being.

Third, and most important of all, though it is part and parcel of the first two, the supporting person can stand by physically and emotionally. Waiting for death is the loneliest time a person can experience. A warm, human contact brings surcease from desolation for a time. Cobb (1962) puts it this way: "Often patients yearn for physical contact, and a touch on the hand or shoulder soothes and reassures the weary wanderer between two worlds" (p. 155).

It is not so much what one says as it is that he is there, and says something that diverts the patient's thoughts to more cheerful topics, or allows the patient to lose himself in the happenings of the day.

If a family member is to become the emotional "Rock of Gibraltar" for the patient, he must have guidance and support. If the husband or wife can talk through approaches with the counselor, some of the anguish is drained off and he or she can meet the needs of the spouse with sensitivity and concern for the patient, rather than anxiety relative to his own grief. A supportive member should always remember to keep the patient involved in the activities of the family. If there is a problem, the patient senses it and may imagine it to be worse than it is. Even a worry over a problem may relieve the nagging anxiety of his illness for a short while, and he feels that he is still an important part of the family.

Sometimes, the family members feel that they must keep a cheerful face regardless. The patient sometimes interprets this false front as indifference. Let the patient know you love him, that you are aware of his pain and his condition, but share with him your "hope that things will be better." Listen to what he has to say; let him talk. It is hard to hear one you love talk about dying or his discouragement, but he needs to talk about his feelings to someone who cares.

The relationship that grows during this sharing of grief and hope is the most beautiful an individual ever experiences. It is the epitomized expression of love. On numerous occasions the husband or wife of a cancer patient, who has lingered for a number of months before death claimed them, communicated with the counselor afterwards to say that the last few months of sharing had been the deepest expression of love and happiness of their marriage. One man said:

> We went home (from the hospital) and I sold our house and bought a trailerhouse. She (the wife) had always talked about seeing the ocean, and the mountains. She was feeling pretty good after treatment, but we both knew and had discussed our knowledge that her days were limited. So we set out to see as many of the things she had dreamed about as we had time to make. We traveled slow and rested a lot. She bloomed. For awhile, it was like she was well again!
>
> We made it. We saw the mountains and we went on over to the ocean side and stayed there for as long as she wanted. She got brown as a berry. Then one day, she said she was ready to come home. We worked our way back another route and both enjoyed it, but we rested more.
>
> Yesterday, we brought her back into the hospital. We both know this is it. But we are so grateful for the most wonderful days of our lives, and we are prepared for whatever comes (Cobb, 1962, Case Notes).

ILLUSTRATIVE MEDICAL AND PSYCHOLOGICAL PROBLEMS SPECIFIC TO TWO DIVERSE CATEGORIES OF CANCER

The preceding sections have dealt with cancer diagnosis and treatment on a general basis. Inasmuch as this disease entity is a multifaceted one, it is deemed helpful to the new counselor, or the family member, to outline specific problems associated with the medical and psychological course of two diverse types of cancer. Because cancer of the head and neck is probably the most mutilating type of cancer, this category has been chosen for presentation. The type that most often involves the younger age group (from ten to thirty years) is cancer of the bone and soft tissues; therefore, a discussion of this category has been included.

Cancer of the Head and Neck

The reported incidence of cancer of the head and neck has increased in the past twenty-five years. It is possible that the incidence has remained stable, but the reporting has improved. This improvement in reporting could be due to improved diagnostic methods, increase in the population, increased longevity of the population, or to the fact that cancer registries are being kept in more hospitals and medical centers than before.

Cancer of the head and neck is probably the greatest ego threat of all malignancies because of its visibility. The disease and its cure are both highly mutilative, and even at best the body image is damaged.

Medical Factors Involved in Treatment of Cancer of the Head and Neck

The primary goal of treatment of malignancies of the head and neck is, of course, cure. The diagnostic process is designed to determine the possibility of cure. Treatment is then planned, in accordance with the diagnosis, to be curative, palliative, or both.

The treatment of choice for cancer of the head or neck is surgery. This involves surgical resection of the primary tumor and regional lymph nodes. This surgery may be followed by irradiation of the primary site, plus regional lymph nodes, or the physician may wish to do irradiation first as indicated by the specifics of the case. A combination, then, of irradiation and surgery may be prescribed. Adjuvant chemotherapy may be used (Healey, 1970).

In this category of cancer, the physician and the patient are interested not only in the cure, but also in functional and cosmetic results as well. This complicates the procedures and the results in that many of the curative and/or palliative procedures produce either functional or cosmetic defects—or both. For example, treatment for cancer of the maxillary sinus may require enucleation of the eye-ball, with partial or total blindness. Radical surgery on the nasal cavity may result in an impairment of the sense of smell. Paralysis of the muscles of the face may follow parotid gland surgery. Removal of the tongue and mandible damages the process of mastication. Cancer of the tongue may result in destruction of taste buds as well as impairment of speech. Removal of the larynx results in loss of speech. If the spinal accessory nerve is severed, movements of the neck and shoulder are limited. In addition to these functional problems, the patient must cope with the accompanying cosmetic disfigurement.

In malignancies of the head and neck, then, the patient must have an important role in decisions of treatment. The physician must first determine the curability or incurability of the case. This is often made by presence or absence of distant metastasis. If the cancer is deemed curable, the patient and his family must not only be made aware of the meaning of the proposed cure in terms of mutilation, but also briefed on possible cosmetic reconstruction available. These choices will often depend on the physician himself and the resources he has available. The age of the patient must be considered as well as the time element involved. Factors such as time for the slow procedures, in terms of remaining lifespan and energy output of the patient, must be weighed. Such procedures are very expensive; therefore, the economic situation of the patient should be considered and the case referred to one of the available research centers where medical care can be provided at no cost or at minimal expense, if the patient so desires.

Often, the pain the patient is experiencing leads him to grasp at any hope for betterment. At times the odor from the fulminating abscesses makes radical surgery acceptable to the patient just to eliminate the sickening smell.

If the case is deemed incurable, the physician and the patient may decide on resection for relief of pain or odor. Irradiation is often prescribed as a palliative measure in such cases.

Psychological Aspects of the Treatment and Course of Cancer of the Head and Neck

Because of the visibility of the mutililation associated with cancer of the head and neck, this type of malignancy, probably more than any other type, poses the greatest emotional threat to the patient and his family. Too often, even with excellent medical care, the patient is left with an eye, part or all of a nose, ear or other portion of the face and neck missing. Despite giant strides in the areas of plastic surgery and prosthetics, the disfigurement is still grossly apparent. It is traumatic to experience mutilation of the body image by loss of a limb, but to endure the agony of a face made grotesque to the point that even friends and family members avert their eyes while speaking with the patient, or betray repulsion in other ways, in excruciating punishment. To live with the knowledge of the presence of foul odors arising from some of the fulminating tumors, and to realize how abhorrent the smell is to others is another step into emotional hell. To lose the ability to speak and be forced to communication in a "Donald Duck" type esophageal speech is psychologically offensive, especially to younger women. The patient needs and deserves the unconditional regard and emotional support of the entire medical team (including an empathic psychiatrist or psychologist), as well as the encouragement of a loving and understanding family.

The psychological services essential to the good mental health of the patient with head or neck cancer will be discussed under three topics. First, the emotional preoperative preparation of the patient and his family will be considered. Second, the psychological reaction to the postoperative disfigurement by the patient, his family, and sometimes his surgeon, will be weighed. And, finally, the special problems posed by the loss of speech will be reviewed.

Psychological Preparation of the Patient for Unavoidable Disfigurement

When the onslaught of the disease process and the results of the treatment essential must result in facial disfigurement, the patient and his family have a right to know the expected extent of the damage. When this knowledge is made known, it would require superior persons to accept the realistic facts without reeling emotionally. In these instances, both the patient and his family need not only the empathic support of his physician, but the opportunity to work through the ego-block with a competent psychiatrist, psychologist, or social worker. They need exact medical information concerning the surgical procedures, what to expect, and what can be done to reconstruct the area mutilated. They need emotional support to work through the depression and real fear of rejection that must arise from the loss. The patient will want to discuss not only his own emotional reactions, but how he can make the impact easier for those he loves.

The family members will need to work through their own repulsive reactions and deep grief in order to protect the patient and make it easier for him. Preparation for treatment includes accurate medical information and hopeful emotional support for both the patient and his family.

Reaction to Disfigurement

No matter how carefully the patient and his family have been prepared for the results of treatment, the accomplished fact is always a shock. To know it will happen is one thing, to live with it is another. The emotional support needed in the early post-treatment days is great. The courage and optimism of many of the patients under the most trying and painful circumstances are humbling.

The physician, the psychiatrist, psychologist, or social worker will be struck with the terrible courage that rises to meet this disaster in many cases. Cobb (1959) speaks of one dauntless woman who continued to operate a village grocery store, with apparent good mental health, even though she had lost one eye, all of her nose, part of one cheek, and her upper lip. She wore a cloth patch over the invaded portion of her face and carried on as if this were the fashion of the day.

Family members also need a listening ear, and someone who can help them learn to accept the damage and rise above their grief. Usually, it is the unconditional acceptance of the patient by his family that makes it possible for him to accept himself, and to seek the acceptance of others in his social world.

One must never forget that the physician, too, is deeply involved in these cases. He entered the profession with the desire to heal, not mutilate. His emotional gratification comes' from cures of disease, not controls. When the cure, or control, leaves a disfigured individual, despite his every effort, the emotional impact on the physician is tremendous. The patient and his family, as well as other members of the medical team, should remember this fact, and also give subtle emotional support and understanding to the doctor in charge.

Special Problems Encountered in Loss of Speech

Removal of the larynx brings about loss of speech. This is a threat to communication that is painful to consider. The patient, however, has three methods of communication left him. He may communicate by hand signals. He may learn esophageal speech, or he may have an artificial larynx installed.

The medical consensus seems to be that every effort should be expended toward the development of esophageal speech (Healey, 1970). Psychologically, the raspy texture of the new voice seems unpleasant to most women patients. Indeed, one younger woman (probably in her early thirties) withdrew into a psychotic episode when a man who spoke esophageal came to talk with her prior to her operation. The intent was to reassure her; the Donald Duck quality of his voice repulsed her.

The psychological significance of the loss of voice could be explored, and preparation for the loss built around this intimate meaning. In the young woman referred to above, the prospect of loss of her natural voice and the acquisition of the raspy sound, was tantamount to loss of sexual attractiveness. When her husband assured her of his love, and when other laryngectomized patients, who spoke more naturally, were brought in (following treatment for the psychotic episode), she was able to face the radical treatment essential to cure of the disease.

Careful medical consideration should be given when the patient is not motivated to attempt esophageal speech, or if the individual is elderly. Improvements in the artificial larynx are needed, but with rapid advancements in biomedical-electronic fields, improvements should be forthcoming, and could solve some of the problems of those who cannot master esophageal speech.

Surgical attempts to create an air tunnel to facilitate speech in the laryngectomized patient have not been entirely successful (Healey, 1970). The development of an artificial larynx, or pseudolarynx, by surgical measures seems to be a new challenge to experimental surgery replacing work on the air tunnel.

Cancers of the Bone and Soft Tissues

In 1968, the American Cancer Society estimated that the incidence of cancer of the extremities ran over nine thousand per year (Healey, 1970). Tumors of bone and soft tissues most commonly involve the younger age group (from ten to thirty years). Bone and soft tissue tumors frequently affect children and adolescents. The overall prognosis of these patients is more guarded than for those with cancer of the breast or thyroid. The variety of tumor types and anatomic sites involved make the rehabilitative process complex.

Medical Factors Involved in Treatment of Cancer of the Bone and Soft Tissues

Cancers of the soft tissues arise from structures such as fibrous tissues, fat, fascia, muscles, tendons, nerves, lymphatics, and vascular structures. Bone cancers develop in any anatomical part of the bone, producing either a bone destruction or the formation of new bone.

Treatment of choice for both soft tissue and bone malignancies is usually surgery. In cancer of the soft tissues when diagnosis is early an "en bloc dissection" (Healey, 1970, p. 85) is recommended. This is a surgical procedure in which large muscle groups are removed, leaving enough limb to be useful to the patient. In many instances, however, amputation is indicated.

Irradiation may be used for palliative purposes when surgery is not feasible. It is sometimes used postoperatively also for palliative reasons.

The treatment of choice for cancer of the bone is also surgery. Following a lower extremity amputation, the major muscle group involved is sewn together over the severed end of the bone. When possible, a three-ply sock is applied, and a rigid plaster-of-paris bandage contoured to the stump. The prosthetic unit is then incorporated into this stump bandage. This unit then receives the temporary pylon which permits ambulation within forty-eight hours (Healey, 1970, p. 86).

Radiotherapy is utilized as an adjunct to surgery. It lessens pain and seems to slow the growth of the malignant cells. It is considered a temporary measure.

Pain in Cancer of Bone and Soft Tissue

Pain is a major problem in bone cancer. Lawrence J. Pool, M.D., Director, Rehabilitation Project, Memorial Sloan-Kettering Cancer Center, New York, has suggested that the two main types of pain encountered in bone cancer are phantom limb pain or awareness, and the painful stump (Healey, 1970). Doctor Pool states that, although all amputees probably experience phantom pain or awareness, only about 3 percent report the sensation. Dr. Pool's explanation of the phantom limb awareness is that the experience results from "upsetting the feedback balance to the cortex and thalamus":

> Nobody knows for sure what the mechanism is, but I think it's the upsetting of the sensory feedback balance to the thalamus and

cortex sensory association areas; not the primary sensory cortex but just beyond it where the sensations are synthesized and put together in a recognizable form. This electrical circuit, if you will, is disturbed by the cutting off of the limb (Healey, 1970, p. 93).

Dr. Pool described a neurological procedure he performed to relieve phantom pain in cancer. The physicians of the Conference on Cancer of the Bone and Soft Tissue (Healey, 1970) were in consensus that neither narcotics nor chordotomy can successfully control phantom limb pain. The use of hypnosis to alleviate intractable pain has been documented by Doctor Miller (Healey, 1970, p. 94).

Doctor Miller also mentioned at the conference the work of a group of anesthesiologists who taped the conversations in the operating room at time of surgery. Six months later, according to this report, the patient would be hypnotized, age-regressed to the time of the operation, and asked to recall the conversation heard during his surgery. Memory recall was checked against the tapes. Recall was phenomenal. As an outcome of this experiment, while the patient was still under anesthesia, he was given the suggestion, "You will not feel any pain." This technique was reported to work in almost 80 percent of the patients. These patients had no need for narcotics following surgery.

Surgeons and psychiatrists (Healey, 1970) agree that the immediate postoperative application of the stump sock and plaster to immobilize the stump for early prosthetic fitting lessens both wound and phantom pain.

The painful stump (neucoma pain) develops in the post-amputation period. This trauma may often be prevented by early proper treatment of the stump. It can also be corrected by a resectioning and capping of the nerve end. This is true nerve pain while the phantom may be due to brain distortion.

Cousalgia results when a nerve is only partially injured. Partial injury to a nerve will induce disturbance of the autonomic system leading to excessive perspiration and vascular changes in the extremity.

Psychological Implications of Loss of an Extremity

Strong emotional stress results from the loss of an extremity. The individual is called upon to give up a part of himself and to modify his body image. This brings into focus fears of pain, of mutilation, of social unacceptability, and of death. Anxiety is present. If the patient is to be able to accept and respond maximally to treatment, these fears and his mourning must be recognized and dealt with.

The anxiety experienced varies with the age of the patient. In the young child, the trauma of the parent must be considered as well as the apprehension of the child. The stress experienced by the adolescent is specific to his stage of development. The adult's concerns are intensified by his apprehension relative to possible impairment of his ability to earn a livelihood, and the emotional reaction to his family, as well as the stress of the financial burden he visualizes. To the older patient the trauma is specific to fears of body deterioration and the burden he may become to his children, or spouse. Each will be reviewed briefly.

When a young child is faced with amputation, the major psychological stress will be experienced by the parents. If the child is seen as an extension of the parents, loss of a limb and threat to his life become a greater stress than the same loss to the parent himself would be. If there has been some ambivalence, or hostility, toward the child on the part of the parent (or parents), guilt reactions are likely. This guilt often results in overprotection of the child and undue demonstrations of love. The anxiety of the parents must be dealt with, or the child will suffer vicariously from their contagious fears. Once the parents have reached some acceptance, the child should be told what to expect. If the parents are mature and loving, they may wish to break the news to their child themselves. If they are not, a relaxed physician, psychiatrist, or psychologist should be called in to perform this service in such a way as to give the child some reassurance and the security of trust in his doctor and parents.

Amputation of an extremity during the adolescent period is probably the greatest blow of all, coming at a time when the ego is particularly sensitive and when the body image is just crystallizing. The young patient may need constant emotional support in order to adapt and rebuild his self-concept. This is a time when youth seeks to be like everybody else in his group.

To suddenly have only one leg, or hand, sets him apart in a damaging way. Often young boys view amputation of a leg as castration. Girls sometimes feel that with a damaged body they will never be able to marry.

On the other hand, adolescents are individuals too, and many times their acceptance of the loss of an extremity is exemplary. Cobb (1959) tells the story of a thirteen-year-old girl who was faced with a hip disarticulation. She had been in considerable pain. The psychologist was requested to talk with her regarding the impending operation. The patient listened intently, asked several questions, was reassured she would be up on crutches and walking in a very few days, and reminded that the removal of the primary tumor would alleviate the pain she was enduring. When the surgeon came by to see her later in the day, he reported (with some emotion) that she reassured him! This patient did walk on crutches a few days postoperatively; she returned to school and, despite the availability of a lifelike artificial limb, continued to use her crutch. It seemed more like her own leg, she said.

When the patient who is to endure an amputation is an adolescent, then care should be taken that the reason for the operation is explained fully. Questions should be carefully answered. The ability to walk, or use of the arm or hand, should be emphasized, and the intelligence and sensitivity of the individual recognized and respected. Most of the time, adolescents will respond beautifully to this adult approach. At the same time, it must not be forgotten that in many ways the adolescent is still a child; so mood swings should be expected and the needs expressed should be met.

The adult man who faces an amputation feels an emotional brunt that is threefold. The first reaction may be one of deep concern at the loss of a limb, and the symbol that loss becomes, of possible impending death. The second impact is so strong that often the first is submerged. "How will this amputation affect my ability to make a living for my family?" he asks himself and the doctor. Financial security for his family has been his major concern through the years; what will happen now? Finally, he wonders how his family will feel about him as a part of a person, rather than a whole. Will they love him and respect him as before? Will he become a financial and emotional burden to them?

These debilitating conflicts must be explored and met, to some extent at least, if the patient is to utilize his energy effectively in getting well.

The mourning at the loss of a part of his body is a natural reaction that he should not be ashamed to express. Once he has explored his feelings about this loss, and has been told by his doctor of his ability to walk again (with crutch or prosthesis), he is ready to move on to coping with the financial problems and the emotions of the family. This is the reason that instant fitting of the prosthesis following surgery is advantageous. The motivation of the patient is provided and maintained by this early effective ambulation.

The pressing financial problems can most effectively be dealt with by the rehabilitative counselor. If he is called in to see the patient even before the surgery, it prevents much anxiety. In fact, he may be able to supplant it with healing hope. The patient is reassured that if he can return to his usual means of earning a living, he will have help to do so. If he finds this impossible, he is told of training and support until he is ready for, and placed in, a new job. This training alone with early ambulation keeps motivation high and depression minimal.

The family reaction to his loss of a limb should be approached first by work with the family members. The patient's condition and prognosis should be discussed by the physician to the point that the family members are aware of the limitations and emotional qualms of the patient.

The rehabilitative counselor may then assist the family in assuming a supportive and reassuring role. If the wife and children do not minimize his loss but make him feel that he is loved, and needed to guide and to provide, the patient seems able to rise above anxiety and pick up the responsibilities and joys of a full life. If the family overprotects him, or leaves him out, they hinder his recovery.

The problems of the working woman facing amputation are very similar to those of the man just discussed. She, however, must also cope with the perceived loss of beauty and femininity at an even deeper level than does the man. Her worth as a woman is threatened. She needs all the emotional support mentioned above plus almost constant (for a while), but subtle, reassurance of her charm and ability to inspire love.

The housewife will experience the same traumas. Her concern will center more around her ability to care for her family, but she will need the same sincere reassurance of the love and understanding of her family and friends.

Amputation in the older patient (65 years and above) seems to reinforce his fear that his body is deteriorating. This fear, of course, leads immediately to thoughts of death, and depression sets in. This depression often is not so much anxiety at approaching death as it is concern for the financial burden he is, or may become, to his children. He may be caught in an ambivalent situation where he, on the one hand, lashes out at this dependency because he has for so long assumed the supportive role.

Here again, the physician and the rehabilitation counselor must work together to interpret the patient to the family, and the family to the patient in such a way as to bring harmony and understanding. Often, the children do not accept, or understand, this changing of the roles. They tend to think of father and mother as always adult, always coping, always equal to any emergency. When they are led to understand that the time has come that mother or dad needs to look to them for protection and comfort, they usually respond. Illness or the amputation may hasten this change of roles. On the other hand, as with the adolescent, the older person is an individual. He may accept the body loss with equanimity, walk in a few days, and return to independent living.

Rehabilitative counselors and family members who work or live with the geriatric patient should read carefully some of the recent research in the area. A panel discussion of medical management, energy conservation, nerves and proprioceptive problems, and rehabilitation of the geriatric population, prepared by the National Research Council's Committee on Prosthetic Research and Development (WHO, 1966), is recommended.

REHABILITATIVE SERVICES IN CANCER

Prior to 1966, the problem of rehabilitation of the cancer patient was more academic than realistic. In the first place, many physicians were still unaware of the availability of rehabilitative services for individuals with malignant disease. Some of those who knew of the agency and its work, because of the uncertainty of the prognosis, failed to refer cancer patients for services. On the agency side, two eligibility requirements made it difficult to accept cancer patients for service. First, to be eligible for rehabilitative services prior to 1967, the client was required to be eighteen months postoperative without evidence of metastasis. Second, feasibility for full-time employment was also a prerequisite for eligibility. Combine these facts with the prevailing feeling of despondency as to the outcome of cancer treatment and it is really surprising that the question of services to the cancer patient even came under discussion.

Recent Developments

However, as the medical world became more and more interested in the quality of survival, and as the improved knowledge and techniques made possible a longer, more comfortable life expectancy for the cancer victims, rehabilitation came into focus. In the meantime, a change in the definition of rehabilitation made full-time employability no longer demanded. Under the new regulations, the client could be served when he had only part-time work potential and/or if she were a housewife. The eighteen-month waiting period was removed.

As the need for services and the vocational potential of the surviving cancer patient were recognized, federal funds were allocated to initiate and carry out services to the cancer patient. Clark and Moreton (Healey, 1970) of the University of Texas M. D. Anderson Hospital and Tumor Institute of Houston, Texas, reviewed the early history of the rehabilitative program there:

However, it was not until 1965 that national legislation established the Regional Medical Programs for Heart Disease, Cancer, and Stroke. Through the efforts of Miss Mary Switzer, legislation made grant funds available in 1966 from the Vocational Rehabilitation

Administration of the Department of Health, Education, and Welfare for the rehabilitation of victims of cancer; interest then began to refocus from the primary concern of five-year survival rates to the possibilities of rehabilitation of these cancer patients (p. 1).

Even with money available and the new mandate on eligibility, the rehabilitation of this new clientele did not progress rapidly. Clark and Moreton explain:

Even after attempts were made to establish programs, as was the case at M. D. Anderson Hospital, the facilities were so fragmented there was often little patient benefit. Adequately trained personnel and space were often not available. Too few of the services, such as the Medical Social Service Department which assisted with socioeconomic problems of the patient and the family, vocational counseling, ministerial and volunteer services, were activities independent of the medical staff.

Other than one or two institutions that had programs oriented toward the physical rehabilitation of the cancer patient, such as Dr. Howard Rusk's program at New York University, initiated in 1946, there were no institutions in the country that were directed toward the total rehabilitation of the cancer patient (p. 1).

M. D. Anderson Hospital did offer a number of rehabilitation services prior to 1966; however, the first program to be established there followed the close of World War II when a war veteran who had lost his larynx was employed to work with laryngectomized cancer patients to teach them to speak again. Eventually, this program became a cooperative venture with the Houston Speech and Hearing Center.

By 1952, a program of maxillofacial and dental restoration for head and neck patients was established through the collaboration of the University of Texas Dental Branch, Rice University, and the University of Houston with M. D. Anderson Hospital. Programs were also initiated to restore shoulder function following radical mastectomy and neck surgery and to prevent the "frozen shoulder syndrome" following preoperative irradiation for breast cancer. Occupational therapy, "which had previously been little more than craftwork, was expanded to include functional therapy and muscle reconditioning particularly of the upper extremities and hands, the design of adaptive equipment to encourage self-help activities, and much attention to the psychological as well as the physical needs of the patient" (Healey, 1970, pp. 2-3).

Paients were not solicited by the rehabilitation personnel of M. D. Anderson Hospital. Referral was strictly at the discretion of the attending physician. . . . In 1960 to 1961 there were 280 new patients referred. . . . In 1966 to 1967 there were 762 new patients referred (Healey, 1970, p. 3).

In 1966, four grants were awarded to M. D. Anderson Hospital to increase cancer rehabilitative services. Neuromuscular effects of drug treatment in pediatric leukemia patients and initiation of early physical restoration for all neurosurgical patients were studied. The Regional Maxillofacial Restorative Center was established to serve a five-state region. Finally orientation and instructional courses for vocational rehabilitation counselors and other ancillary personnel were conducted by the hospital staff. Also during that year, a cooperative program to expedite early postoperative fitting of prostheses for cancer patients undergoing limb amputation was initiated with the Texas Institute for Rehabilitation and Research.

Since 1966, all rehabilitative programs at M. D. Anderson Hospital have been centralized under the direction of Dr. John E. Healey, Jr., in the Department of Rehabilitation Medicine. Under his leadership, a comprehensive rehabilitative center for cancer patients is to be opened in late 1972: "It will provide medically-supervised housing and vocational rehabilitation for the patients who no longer need to occupy a hospital bed but are not yet ready to return to their communities, or who require ambulatory therapy" (Healey, 1970, p. 5).

Future Availability of Services

Despite the more liberal rehabilitative eligibility policies, a number of problems still prevent adequate service coverage of the cancer cases. First, attending physicians are still predominantly unaware of, or indifferent to, the availability of rehabilitative services. Second, the medical prognosis is still quite guarded. Third, when a patient is referred, the rehabilitative counselor is still uncertain of the vocational feasibility of the client. He needs much more information relative to the disease process and treatment as well as experience and research in effective placement of these clients. Finally, and this is probably the most urgent factor, there is the need of the prospective employers of controlled or cured cancer patients for information as to the life expectancy and vocational potential of these individuals.

It would seem, then, that improved rehabilitative services are dependent in great measure on comprehensive educational programs. First, and perhaps foremost, is the education of the physician himself. Healey (1970) states: "When medical students and physicians are better informed regarding the value an availability of rehabilitative measures, more progress can be anticipated in the field of rehabilitation" (p. 169).

A second, challenging, educational goal is the dissemination of correct information to the public. Much effort has been, and is being expended in this direction. More emphasis should be placed on the rehabilitative potential of the cancer patient. When the public becomes aware of the need and the availability of services, pressure will be exerted that will produce more effective procedures, and more referrals.

The family constellation is another important target area for cancer education. The major emotional support to the patient and cooperative agent to the physician is the family. In order to be of maximum assistance to the patient and to the medical team in the treatment effort, the family must have accurate and complete information relative to the disease process and the treatment employed. The busy physician may not have time to instruct each family group personally. He should, however, arrange for adequate written or verbal instruction to insure the emotional support of his patient. Written information should be prepared by professionals under medical guidance. Verbal instructions and support could be given the family by experienced social workers, nurses, psychologists, or rehabilitative counselors, again working in collaboration with the attending physician. This one educational area could result in significant improvements in the emotional and career rehabilitation of cancer patients.

Finally, the patient himself has tremendous educational needs. He needs to know the what's, how's and why's of each phase of his treatment. His education should begin upon diagnosis and during the pre-treatment phase. Throughout the treatment period he must have continued instruction and emotional support. After treatment, if the disease is under control, he needs reassurance and assistance in reestablishing his career. If the disease is deemed incurable, the patient needs added information as to the final stages of the disease process, and emotional support to come to grips with the encounter with death.

The closing comments of the Proceedings of Three Interdisciplinary Conferences on Rehabilitation of the Patient with Cancer summarized the critical medical challenge yet to be met in the rehabilitation of the cancer patient (Healey, 1970):

> It was the consensus that the medical profession should alter its concept of cancer. We should emphasize the successes, rather than the failures as we have in the past. We should take a positive approach in handling and controlling, as well as curing this disease. The cancer patient should be regarded in the same way as any patient who is afflicted with a chronic disease. We need not always wait for a cure before starting rehabilitation measures. . . . We must develop a positive, hopeful and eventually successful outlook among the medical profession as well as the public in dealing with all aspects of the disease—cancer (p. 184).

The vocational rehabilitative challenge in cancer is just as critical as the medical. So little is known of the work-related problems of the cancer patient as he returns to employment. Much action research through carefully planned experience will help to open the world of work to these clients. The rehabilitative counselor's knowledge of the course and results of treatment for this disease is far too limited. Expanding educational endeavors on the part of cancer research and treatment centers will bridge that gap. Continued efforts to make employers aware of the work potential of cancer patients will lead to greater acceptance, not only of the disease but also of the client in the business world. The greatest challenge of all lies in the preparation and support of the patient and his family as they face the diagnosis, treatment, control and/or the knowledge of the incurability of the disease.

Doctor Healey (1970) said it beautifully, quoting a participant of a concerence: "The first principle of rehabilitation, I believe is not to be satisfied with life-saving but to be equally as concerned with the quality of living and not merely the quantity of the not-yet dead" (p. v).

Doctors Clark and Moreton (Healey, 1970) spoke of rehabilitation as opening "a door long closed to the cancer patient. To give these patients hope for a useful remaining life is a worthy goal" (p. 5). The quality of survival—this is the goal and the challenge of rehabilitation in cancer today.

REFERENCES

Clark, Randolph Lee and Cumley, Russell W.: *The Year Book of Cancer.* Chicago, Year Book Publishers, 1957.

Cobb, A. Beatrix: Cancer. In Garrett, James F. and Levine, Edna S. (Eds.): *Psychologcal Practices with the Disabled.* New York, Columbia U Pr, 1962.

Cobb, Beatrix: Emotional problems of adult cancer patients. *J Am Geriatr Soc,* 7:274-283, no. 2, 1959.

Cobb, Beatrix: Psychological impact of long illness and death of a child on the family circle. *J Pediatr, 49*:746-751, no. 6, 1956.

Dorland, W. A. Newman: *Medical Dictionary,* 23rd ed. Philadelphia, Saunders, 1957.

Healey, John E., Jr. (Ed.): *Ecology of the Cancer Patient.* Washington, D.C.. The Interdisciplinary Communication Associates, Inc., 1970.

Kuehn, Paul G.: *Quality of Survival of the Cancer Patient.* Hartford, The American Cancer Society (Connecticut Division), 1969.

Stehlin, John S., Jr. and Beach, Kenneth H.: Psychological aspects of cancer therapy, a surgeon's viewpoint. *JAMA, 197*:100-104, July 1966.

World Health Organization Expert Committee: *Cancer Treatment, Report of a WHO Expert Committee.* Geneva, WHO Technical Report Series, no. 322, 1966.

Chapter 3

PSYCHOTHERAPEUTIC WORK WITH THE CANCER PATIENT*

H. H. Garner

The Initial Interview
Brief Psychotherapy
Confrontation Problem-solving Psychotherapy
References

Psychotherapy theory, principles, methods and applicability must be understood as applied generally before its specific applications to a select population, such as cancer patients, are undertaken. Nevertheless, what is written about psychotherapy as it applies generally will be found applicable to the broad spectrum of challenges to one's therapeutic competence with the cancer patient.

Before psychotherapy became established as a word meaning purposeful treatment through communication, healers had unknowingly been using it as their major agent for healing. The degree of authority with which instructions and management procedures are carved out has healing virtues, at least in so far as any or all of them met the needs of the patient. Most of the circumstances surrounding the physician-patient relationship, even instrumentation, have significant psychological meaning.

* I wish to acknowledge the contributions of Dr. John Cowen, Professor of Psychiatry and Behavioral Sciences of the Chicago Medical School, for editing and developing the content of some of my original work.

For this reason, a number of techniques constantly used has to be listed as of psychotherapeutic virtue. For example, ordering a patient to take his insulin injections twice daily is effective only insofar as he accepts the implicit injunction that it is preferable to stay alive and that this depends on the insulin effect. The success following the advice of a three-month stay in Arizona may not be due so much to the inhalation of unpolluted air as to being away from a stressful interaction with the family. One recalls the avidity and success with which some rheumatic patients thirty years ago drank a vivid blue suspension of aspirin powder, while contemptuous of the virtue of the much cheaper regular tablets.

Psychotherapeutic measures are believed to be generally, although by no means always, only temporarily efficacious, for they are often effective by suppression, or by evasion, of problems. In the cancer patient, the acceptance of a solution suggested by a respected therapist may be desirable. However, in the technique to be later described, the objective is to help by exposing the problems, and showing how the patient himself may set about their solution, provided that he can be led into a mature relationship. The former approaches are often referred to as supportive forms of psychotherapy because to a very large extent the healing process is related to the degree of dependence which is fostered and permitted to develop in the treatment situation.

THE INITIAL INTERVIEW

The first interview has therapeutic potential. The seed of that relationship which will influence the future mutuality of feeling, confidence, trust, respect, and empathy is implanted. The interview can also be the first psychotherapeutic meeting.

In all our relationships with other human beings, intellectual perception of them and their setting is barren unless it is accompanied by emphatic emotional attitudes. In the therapist-patient relationship, too, intellectual understanding is inadequate unless it is also accompanied by an emotional appreciation. Only when a patient feels the therapist to be reliable, trustworthy, and genuinely interested will he understandingly permit exposure of anxiety-laden material. The therapist must listen not only to objective statements but also to undertones revealing covert feelings.

The initial interview is a primary technical procedure. Regardless of the type of illness, one should apply psychologic, biological, and social knowledge to the understanding of individuals, as members of a family, and of specific social groups.

The aims of an interview diverge somewhat, and the lines of inquiry become directed along two channels. One line of inquiry is concerned with socioenvironmental factors. The therapist must ask himself, "What noxious agents, objects, conditions, or people cause this person to be ill? In what way? How can it be altered?" Another line of inquiry concerns the patient himself, the influences of his personality, and somatic reactions. Here, one tries to answer the question, "What is his reaction to the noxious influences? Is the situation *necessarily* noxious? Is his perception or reaction trend noxious? How can my knowledge of his personality be utilized to improve his care and his favorable reaction to that care?"

The interview situation is in essence an interpersonal relationship and the therapist is one of the two human beings comprising it. He possesses unconscious as well as conscious motivations, prejudices, and objective and subjective reasons for feelings and behavior. Toward almost every bit of information, the therapist may have developed certain preconceived attitudes and the assumption that only his attitudes are correct. For a successful interview, it is essential that he refrain from imposing these judgments. He must learn to counteract the tendency to criticize or derogate behavior which deviates from his personal standards. In all but a few exceptional instances, he must be free of authoritarian attitudes and autocratic behavior. Real acceptance means accepting the feelings expressed. It does not necessarily involve acceptance of unsocial behavior. Attempts to deny or suppress one's own feelings may result in artificial, stilted responses. It is better to recognize feelings for what they are. They need not be shared. Control, rather than absence, of feeling is the desirable goal.

Accusatory questions, or those with hostile implications arouse fear, suspicion, or anger and do not inspire cooperation. The interviewer should carry his inquiry only as far as necessary and still be effective. A good general rule is to question for one of two purposes: (1) to obtain specifically needed information, or (2) to direct the conversation from fruitless into fruitful channels.

The first and last sentences uttered are often of unusual significance. The manner in which a problem is stated always bears special study, since it reveals a key to hidden problems and the attitude toward seeking help. Often a last remark indicates either a summing up of what the interview has meant, or the degree to which forces have been mobilized for working out his problem.

Previous knowledge concerning the patient's feelings about personal appearance may make slight change in clothing necessary, such as putting on or taking off a coat, refraining from or proceeding to smoke, whichever might better aid in establishing rapport at the outset.

One does not reveal significant, emotionally charged data unless one senses real interest and increased, appreciative understanding with each revelation.

Gestures are often needed to draw out people. They need not be elaborated or contrived, but rather, the conventional evidences of human interest—sympathetic facial expressions, a warm tone of voice, an occasional word of encouragement. To be effective, one need not talk a great deal, but one must be alert to what is said. From time to time, appropriate questions may be used to stimulate the flow of thoughts, but generally, permitting the story to unfold is the best method to avoid inconsistencies and misunderstandings arising from suggestibility. One should avoid arguing. Persons with chronic, obscure diseases may place uncomplimentary interpretations on any negative interest shown toward their personal reactions. The therapist should be restrained and discreet in offering reassurance. Should the patient become tearful and self-defensive, overtly seeking sympathy, one can point out favorable factors which might encourage and offer hope for a relatively good prognosis. In remarks concerning success in conquering his problem, it is well that answers to questions be pointed and specific as to detail. Any generalized encouraging statement can be disheartening to a person who fails to perceive anything favorable about his condition. Pep talks are frequently depressing. If helpful, they fail progressively on repetition.

The confidential nature of the relationship must indeed be earned. The therapist should never engage in discussions about patients, and should especially avoid depreciating those previously seen. Seemingly innocent, casual remarks about others cause a patient to become resistive and suspicious. "What does he say about me?" The therapist should be discreet, and curb the impulse toward any unnecessary betrayal of confidences. The patient may endow the therapist with negative characteristics. Because he, himself, feels anxious, insecure, and deprived, he may build up antagonism toward the therapist who betrays none of these attributes. Negative feelings may be easily concealed under the cloak of polite social usage. These are more often revealed, however, by refusal to return and sometimes by displaced anger against hospital or office personnel.

Establishing a relationship of truthworthiness and showing a real respect for a person is the core of the psychotherapeutic process. The initial interview may very well bring to the fore reactions based on doubts about the person offering help. Prior negative experiences with significant people or doubts about his own acceptability will be the important factors in his questioning the sincerity of the examiner.

One can say in very general terms that any activity which may with some justification be perceived as evidence of insufficient trustworthiness, respect, or consideration must be dealt with to diminish the patient's hostility toward the therapist. If one takes notes, it may be viewed as the creation of a file of damaging evidence, of failing to be attentive in order to obtain a good record, or of being concerned with facts and material for some ulterior purpose like teaching or research rather than in the patient as a person. Failure to take notes may be similarly interpreted as indifference—"How can you remember these things about me?"—or as carelessness—"You are not even trying to remember." He may feel, however, that the interviewer in not taking notes possesses some unusual gift to remember everything and consequently an unusual gift to cure. Notes, recording of an interview, and other means of making a record supposedly for teaching and research purposes may mobilize megalomanic wishes to have some immortal place in the healing arts and sciences. This by no means exhausts the possible perceptual distortions in this bit of activity.

A sharp and critical eye and ear are needed to note the distortion of the significance of the activity. The therapist should be able to share the realistic basis of his reasons for doing what he is doing about some aspect of the production and behavior. Clarification of the need to distort the real significance of note-taking or the absence of note-taking, of recording or failure to record, will minimize the distortion of such activities in the interpersonal relationship.

Threats, punishment, and disapproval are parental reactions which a person may anticipate. By being a "good patient" he diminishes the risk of punishment and disapproval and enhances the probability of recovery. Expectations are influenced by the nature of the immediate illness, the current problems in living, the level of sophistication, the family and social values, the total personality of the patient, and the personality of the therapist.

The personality of the therapist is an integral factor in the effects produced by all his treatment devices, whether additive, subtractive, or manipulative. Flexibility is an essential quality. Rigidity and an unyielding nature, a preference for an intellectual approach as though the patient were an object, and the avoidance of involvement in the patient's emotional problems are qualities which significantly influence treatment—too often favorably.

A therapist may identify with the patient. He is, for example, often stirred deeply through identification with the dying. His desire not to be reminded of a previous traumatic experience may prevent an attitude of empathy which would be helpful in management. The undesirability of positive identification, as if the individual were a close personal friend or an intimate associate, has been sufficiently stressed.

Authoritarianism is a part of every relationship with a sick person. The patient often needs and expects a certain degree of control. Strong feelings of passivity and dependency drive many patients to extract a maximal degree of authoritarian control and to avoid taking responsibility for self-management and self-control. They will react with anxiety and undesirable behavior if their needs are not recognized.

Obsequiousness toward persons in a prestige relationship may prevent development of the relationship needed for therapeutic effectiveness. It creates a situation in which the sick determine the therapeutic prodecure.

When passive, dependent traits are manifested by the therapist, an atmosphere of doubt is created about the wisdom of his therapeutic procedure. Some patients with anxiety about retaliatory aggressiveness on the part of the therapist may, however, respond to treatment administered by the more passive type of person with greater comfort.

Interviewers are sometimes troubled by personal questions. There are many overt and unconscious motives which prompt such a question. A female asks if the therapist is married before she would venture any revelations about her sexual organs. Or one may be asked, "Are you an M.D.?" lest there be no purpose otherwise in discussing a physical complaint. In most instances, a brief, truthful answer should be given. Attention is redirected to the patient by an interest in the meaning of his question and the effect of the answer.

The universal quest for certainty has a special poignancy. It is present in the person seeking help, whether for a threatening physical disorder or an emotional upheaval. The treatment situation creates certain basic desires which Masserman (1953) has described as essential defenses. In essence, the defenses are (1) a feeling of indestructibility; (2) a client's belief that others are interested in him, even to the point of great personal sacrifice, and (3) faith in some force or power, omnipotent and all-knowing, which in some way will protect him against danger. The therapist as a representative of some significant figure from past experience is utilized to establish the essential defenses. Awareness of the need for such defenses to help protect against anxiety or fear should be part of every therapist's knowledge.

Parallel with the patient's quest for certainty is the therapist's comparable quest. The theory of parsimony invites us all to seek the "one" cause for a situation, thereby implying that there is one treatment which, by eliminating that cause, will inevitably engineer "complete cure." The sick believe this as much as do their therapists who have been exposed to such an indoctrination. While we recall only too easily that there is only one solution for x in a simple equation, its value will differ in quadratic equations.

The senses by which man perceives properties are known to be deceptive; they vary in validity according to needs, preferences, emotions, and state of health. The perceptions are also altered by the morals and culture of the time, and the symbolic values with which the object is endowed. The quest for certainty is the quest for an illusion. The patient's quest for certainty and his need for someone to help him even at a personal sacrifice distorts the image of the healer when patient is experiencing pain, distress, anxiety, or fear.

Transference is the term most commonly used to describe distortion of the healer-patient relationship in psychotherapy. Rapport, confidence, acceptance, empathy, relationships, and many other terms are used to symbolize that interpersonal reaction which characterizes the contractual involvements of treatment. These phenomena are seen and can be studied as elements in any system in which one person seeks help and another offers help. The term "transference" has been used most frequently to designate the special nature of the relationship in psychoanalytic therapy. Treatment has begun the moment a person has decided to seek the help of another. It encompasses the establishment of a relationship of dependency and the revival of the earlier attitudes experienced as a child when continuous protection, care, help, and nourishment as a dependent were needed to maintain life and enable growth. In treatment, many perceptions express this need to see in the therapist the protecting or neglecting, the caring or the injuring roles of significant figures in his past. The response to the therapist may resemble that given to a father, mother, brother, sister, uncle, aunt, teacher, or best friend. This repetitive tendency throughout life is an extension of the principle involved in the behavior of any organism—repetition of the adaptive patterns which earlier had been operationally successful.

Infants and children endow parents with God-like magical powers when they are frightened, in pain or distress, or in any way insecure, and they find that parental intervention restores them to comfort and joy. These same attitudes, expectations, and powers are transferred in later life to the transactions with the therapist. Such reactions are a necessary psychologic aspect of the healing process; sometimes, unfortunately, the therapist accepts at face value what is believed about him.

The most commonly expressed transference attitudes and feelings are the following:

(1) Dependency needs, mobilized by stress of any kind, may be expressed realistically as a dependence appropriate to the disability with recognition of the probable limits of a competent therapist's abiilty to help. At the opposite extreme, these needs may be expressed unrealistically even to the extent of creating th expectation that the therapist will give up his own interests in selfless devotion and accomplish what is beyond the realm of currently known medical science. The patient may remain in bed seeking special attention for the functions of eating, and of bowel and bladder evacuations. Dependency craving may be relatively minor, even ceremoniously proper at first, like enjoying breakfast in bed on Mother's Day, but may be encouraged to merge into the acceptable social role of illness which ultimately may reach a stage of regression that is malignant and non-reversible.

(2) Denial of dependency is a defensive bravado, an ignoring of anxiety. Such a defense may suddenly collapse into a state of acute panic or severe regression to the surprise of all who accepted the defense at face value. The sick person weakened by illness, harried by anxiety, and beset with other problems in the family may alternate feelings and attitudes of dependency with denial of dependency.

(3) Feelings of anger, resentment, and open hostility may

be mobilized by unrealistic expectations. The sick person sees himself as being treated with less consideration or thoroughness than others, or even negligently and incompetently. And the relationship is used to fortify a feeling of basic distrust about any interest or attention shown.

(4) Feelings of guilt may be manifestations of hostile and aggressive intentions.

(5) Erotic feelings and shame may be aroused. Interest especially with regard to the erogenous zones, may be interpreted as having an erotic motivation, and may arouse reactive feelings of anger and shame with accompanying physiologic and behavioral changes.

(6) Feelings of envy and jealousy occasionally interfere with a realistic relationship. The patient may feel that others may be getting better or special treatment.

(7) Anxiety and fear, relative to anticipated punishment or withdrawal of approval, may be aroused.

Therapeutic interventions are seen as powerful, magical controls which are mobilized to help the patient. The willingness to intervene is interpreted as an expression not only of healing power, but also of interest, protection, and love. More latent are concerns about a possible malevolent use of these powers as expressions of anger and hate.

Knowledge of self, so important in the treatment of individuals with emotional illness, is applicable in all treatment. The therapist needs to face maturely any strong feelings of like or dislike. In his devotion to his calling, he may have to discount at times disliking the things he has to do. He must have some measure of charity and tolerance for the foibles, weaknesses, and prejudices of mankind. One's previous personal experiences contribute to one's attitudes.

Countertransference is a term used for the therapist's reaction to the patient with feelings and attitudes similar to those which he had manifested toward significant persons in his past. The feelings and attitudes may reflect the patient's feelings of transference toward the therapist.

Feelings of countertransference are to be distinguished from those which are reasonable, realistic, and appropriate to the circumstances. A patient may be excessively demanding, rude and improper in his speech, manner, and dress, or in other ways behave unacceptably and offensively. He expects that the therapist will, as a human being, react to such behavior with nonacceptance. On the other hand, a therapist's function in society realistically requires that he manifest a tolerant, noncondemning reaction. The degree to which he can be objective and react with understanding, rather than with anger, impulsiveness, and retaliatory or overtly aggressive behavior is a measure of his awareness of his role in society and the maturity of his relationship to patients.

In the seemingly indifferent patient who may be too withdrawn to care, patience may overcome the unconscious expectation that his revelations may overwhelm the listener. The most difficult and anxiety-provoking event for a therapist is to have to sit with a silent patient, particularly at a first interview—for then one has no past pattern by which to gauge the impasse. Prodding only reveals the examiner's mounting anxiety. The patient responds by feeling "If just my presence here makes this man so upset, how much more so will he become if I start talking!"

If little or no exchange occurs, it has to be made clear that reluctance to talk is both understood and accepted; that there is no great hurry; that there can be a second appointment when another meeting will take place; and that if there is a need for help, the availability remains as before. There should be no parting on a sour note.

BRIEF PSYCHOTHERAPY

Psychotherapy is a technique of nonphysical treatment in which the healer offers help to produce beneficial changes in a patient disabled to a lesser or greater degree by emotional conflicts. The intent is to influence feeling, cognition, and behavior so as to bring about a correction in ineffectual living, or relief from suffering, or both. The help rendered is *not* a direct result of any drug administered, nor of any instrument used, with the avowed intention of producing physiologic or anatomic change.

Brief psychotherapy is used to designate a type of one-to-one relationship of a therapist and patient in which the model forty-five to fifty minutes four to five times per week, of psychoanalysis, are replaced by a therapeutic relationship of lesser duration of treatment time and of shorter individual visits.

A visit may vary from a few minutes to several hours. Regularity of time, place and length of time are to be seen as significant rituals which are characteristic for establishing the a helper-to-helped relationship in our culture. There is no reason to believe that brief contacts are incompatible with effective therapy. Much can be accomplished with a few brief visits when goals are limited. Some individuals show a propensity for taking something out of a few brief contacts and going on to significant changes in attitude and behavior. Whether such changes are significant as evidence of compliance or because of more effective coping or adaptive behavior is pertinent to the therapeutic goals. For the cancer patient, ten- to fifteen-minute sessions are often effective and may be the span of time most desirable.

Elements of importance in the initial interview include not only those already mentioned but also those elements considered tools used in the psychotherapeutic work. The initial interview is the first psychotherapeutic effort and in subsequent interviews, a greater or lesser use of the basic tools may be seen.

The tools of psychotherapy are simply the verbal or nonverbal cues intended to convey the messages which are related to exposing the disability and encouraging the reparative process.

Nonverbal Communications

Bodily movement, gestures, and facial expression are tools of communication which can act in concert with, or independently of, verbal tools. They may be conscious as in moving the chair forward to hear better, yet also unconscious of a desire to get closed. He may proclaim no particular emotional impact about a recounted event while displaying dilated pupils, generalized tremors and beads of sweat on the upper lip.

Selective attention is, in short, a prerequisite to the formulation of the selective question which is the safest and most productive form of intervention.

The posing of a question is therefore a well-considered activity which interlocks smoothly into the theme of the individual session. This, too, will be something to listen for as therapy advances: the theme of the session— usually one topic or a series of closely related topics to which frequent referral is made, often rarely consciously.

Trying hard to avoid seduction into the role preset for him by the patient, it may well be difficult for the therapist to avoid slipping into one or more of several interventions considered therapeutic. Often this is a source of secret joy to the patient and bewilderment to the therapist. There may be a place for a single interjection with the intent of suggestion, reassurance, abreaction, persuasion, or clarification. But, as with every intervention, its use has to be well considered, appropriate, and not likely to muddy the stream which has been encouraged to flow.

Selective inattention to physical symptoms—listening with a minimum of evidence to the patient that "he thinks this is so important"—and indirect questioning about symptoms will tend to enhance the treatment relationship. Selective attention to the patient's experiences, events, or emotionally disturbing circumstances tell about how he is living and about his personality and behavior and will encourage an understanding of the problems of life and the desirabiilty of looking for solutions through methods other than the "sick role."

A *listening, noncondemning, nonjudgmental attitude* is basic for the visits. Being humane and patient, having a realistic (humble) opinion about one's importance, yet being capable of recognizing the need to endow the therapist with God-like qualities are essential to effective psychotherapeutic work. When communication proceeds freely, few if any interventions are necessary. The visit might start with "How have you been?" "What is in your mind?" and end with "It seems your main trouble was your husband," or it may end with "You look well; I will see you tomorrow."

Sharpening the technical tools utilized for assimilating information will take place as the therapist learns more about his most valuable therapeutic agent—the patient's actual evaluation and his fantasies about the therapist.

Listening to the patient is not just a passive exercise displaying politeness, patience, and sympathy. A good bartender can do that. Listening has the specific purpose of putting together what is said and what carefully skirts the issues. This is all part of selective attention. When the patient is evidently avoiding an emotionally charged issue, the therapist might wonder out loud why "you don't seem too comfortable talking about what goes on with your daughter . . . husband."

One listens for what is said and for what is almost said. Of equal importance is to listen for the theme which the client is unwittingly trying to convey. The preoccupation may not be ready for immediate exposure. It usually reveals itself, however, in recurring comments and veiled allusions. Not only are these useful clues to the presenting subsurface problem, but they can be used to get back to the topic if he suddenly becomes circumstantial or irrelevant.

ASKING QUESTIONS. When the initial interviewing stage has been left behind, the use of a question can have more signifiance than merely obtaining information. Such comments as (1) tell me about that; (2) how did it happen? (3) give me more of the facts about the situation; (4) describe the details of the incident, or even just nodding and listening will lead to further information. This information usually improves the knowledge and understanding by the therapist in many significant areas: (1) psychogenetically important past experiences, (2) factors which tend to precipitate conflicts, and (3) the manner in which the person is conducting himself in interpersonal relationships with his family and friends at work and at play. The intent is to establish a factual base for the improvement of therapeutic planning.

The questions can also be seen as intended to encourage the

process of, and to further the work of, psychotherapy through exploration, ventilation and clarification, with such comments by the therapist as "Why?" "For instance . . ." "How did you feel about it?" or "How do you feel about it?"

"What could there be about what happened that would upset you?"

—"that would cause you to be afraid?"
—"that would cause you to be angry?"
—"that would annoy you?"
—"that would make you feel it was too much for you?"

These represent but a sample of potential questions.

Sometimes, the patient infers from the questioning some special interest in certain aspects of his life. He may then try to please by giving a voluminous amount of material on that subject. Or the question may be considered an unnecessary, intrusive, and improper probing. When recognized and accepted as it should be intended, namely, as an invitation to further collaborative exploration, the question will tend to stimulate a desire to seek motivations and hidden factors and may lead to illumination of certain disturbing or unacceptable ideas and acts. In this sense, questioning may be found to have the effect of increasing self-observing and self-experiencing tendencies, a process which is considered essential to achieving the goals of psychotherapy.

ELABORATION ON WHAT THE PATIENT DOESN'T SAY OR HASN'T SAID. Shame, guilt, or pride may act to minimize the expression of thoughts and feelings which would add to understanding of the discomfort and could act as a therapeutic, cathartic and ventilating experience if encouraged by appropriate questions. Asking "Was there something about the closeness of your relationship to your friend that troubled you?" may bring a flood of material dealing with guilt feelings about one's hostility. The tendency to circumstantiality, a shy discussion of a subject, an illusion to "what's the use of it all," are examples of the cues which may be detected and may require elaboration on what is not being said. The appropriate questioning adds another dimension to the therapeutic work—catharsis and ventilation in a noncondemning atmosphere diminish anxiety—makes realistic evaluation possible, and therefore, encourages problem-solving thinking.

INQUIRING INTO DAILY ACTIVITIES. Many therapists at some time or other in the course of treatment inquire into the daily activities. The inquiry usually follows some discussion in which a dissatisfaction with inability to do things, with boredom, with lack of interest in the usual day-to-day happenings has been expressed. In general, the patient has indicated a lack of organization and interest in his daily life. The therapist responds because of the generally accepted feeling that activity in social functions or being busy is good for one's mental health. Therapeutic regimens such as the total push method, emphasis on milieu therapy in the hospital setting and similar plans for an ordered activity are mentioned as part of treatment programs. When the therapist inquires into the daily activities, the responses are usually an expression of doubt as to the desirability of being constantly busy, seeking approval for being appropriately busy, or seeking guidance for daily activity programs.

The asking of questions that stem from personal needs of the therapist requires understanding. When the patient is silent, the therapist may be the first one to feel uncomfortable. He may become restless, and find it necessary to intervene much as one does in the strained silence of a social situation. Curiosity, irritation, or frustration press the therapist into taking the initiative. Questioning to the point of probing with some manifestations of a sadistic overtone may occasionally be recognized in the activity. Such interventions need self-understanding and constraint. They can realistically hurt and embarrass, adding unnecessarily to already existing, strong feelings of guilt, inadequacy and hostility.

One may say about asking questions that it encourages the client to think and see relationships for himself. Ultimately he may learn to ask himself the questions which will promote his own problem-solving thinking.

GAPS. Careful listening may reveal gaps in continuity: a skipping, for example, between important biographical events. Usually this indicates some emotional importance attaching to the incident which has been suppressed. If it becomes apparent that without assistance, the gap is going to be left, a comment is in order to request more information about that period. A sudden shift in topic should not be immediately corrected. It should be allowed to develop, for it usually reveals itself to be no real shift, but a continuation of the theme in another guise. A change in talk from home to hospital may still be no change because the theme remains one of resistance to authority.

EARLIEST RECOLLECTIONS. Sometimes almost casually, patients reveal their earliest recollections. These must be picked up by an attentive ear. Although at first hearing they may have no connection with the presenting symptoms, sooner or later they will reveal themselves as important in understanding the basic dynamic structure of the personality. A first memory of a present given at the fifth birthday by a woman housekeeper opened up a vista of understanding about a man who felt that his mother had really given him nothing. Even a poor cleaning woman recognized his needs more than his own mother; or perhaps his mother was in fact poorer than the cleaning woman—so why did she hire help?—was she really sick? The multiple conflicts, both real and in fantasy, which plagued the relationship between this man and his mother from his infancy until her death, and his immediate subsequent depressive attack, can be forecast from this "first memory."

REASSURANCE. Reassurance is intended to describe a special type of activity which is supposedly directed at alleviating anxiety, giving moral support to a viewpoint or action, suggesting and directing channels of behavior and attitudes which correct a fault, diminish the need for guilt feelings and encourage constructive realistic achievement.

Frequently in the first visit, or during a therapy session and often at the end of the visit, a response from the therapist as to the possibility of being helped or of the therapist being able to help is requested. "Can I be helped?" he asks, or "Can you help me?" Such requests for reassurance may be effectively managed by a question from the therapist, "You apparently have doubts about what can be done for you. I wonder why."

Reassurance may essentially confirm the persons own ideas

about the lack of seriousness of his condition, about which he does have a lingering miniscule of doubt. Reassurance removes the doubt because it comes from someone with superior knowledge and status. Experiences have taught the professional that, in similar cases, treatment has been effective in the past, and there is every reason to believe it will be so again.

Reassurance may be offered indirectly by questioning the need to have doubts—e.g. "You seem to find it necessary to depreciate your ability at work. I wonder why."

EXPLANATIONS AND PERSUASION. Explanation and persuasion represent efforts to change a way of behaving or of feeling by the use of what is believed to be logic. For example, "The x-ray plates show quite clearly that you have no ulcer; there is therefore no cause for you to have stomach pains after meals." Or, "Your son died after having led a very contented and successful life; it is time you gave up mourning his death."

Emotions by definition are not governed by reason. The fact that persuasion does seem to be effective is often a consequence of the same influences which adhere to reassurance and to suggestion: magical expectations and hope.

SUGGESTION. Suggestion invokes by direct or indirect command an uncritical compliance in the client. Change of behavior or of perception according to the demand of the therapist is reflected in compliance. It involves the implantation into another, without appeal to his reason, of an idea not acted upon until the cue to act is given by another person.

It is the essential psychic force of magic whereby one can influence another often with what are, in themselves, of course, ineffectual intermediaries. The wand and the potion and the abracadabra are embellishments which distract the subject from what is really going on, namely submission to the control of another.

Even in these days of scientific medicine, much healing is accelerated by the suggestion with which treatment is prescribed and administered. The placebo has "cured" many complaints. A well-fed middle class which nevertheless has vitamin tablets at the table is sufficient proof of the power of suggestion. Television advertising is the supreme example of attempting to influence by deliberate indirect suggestion. It implies that smoking the right brand, using the right deodorant or hair spray, or buying the right car, will ensure greater happiness, usually by making the purchaser sexually irresistible.

The psychotherapeutic intent may be one of bringing about compliance. This having been seen as a reasonable goal in the therapeutic management, then statements that the client agrees to what he has been told, persuaded to accept, commanded to do, or forbidden to carry out, are made frequently.

HYPNOSIS. Hypnosis can be regarded as the ultimate state of suggestion and differs from it in that the former is usually accompanied by some degree of imposed waning in level of consciousness. An atmosphere is set up to induce drowsiness in a subject whose critical faculty is thereby impaired, thus rendering him all the more readily susceptible to suggestion. Hypnosis with trance induction is seldom used in the elderly. Suggestive influences are best understood by seeing the relationship to hypnosis as a therapeutic intervention.

There is as yet no scientific explanation for what is happening in the hypnotic state.

Basic to its production is a necessary combination of a sense of self-confidence on the part of the operator with a willingness to submit on the part of the subject. The suggestibility of the latter varies, as has been said, with the degree of his wakefulness and also with the condition of his general health, his cultural background, influence of drugs he may have taken, the environment in which the procedure is taking place, and his psychological needs at the moment.

The hypnotic state facilitates the implantation of suggestions. Sometimes, and probably because it implies always a diminution in conscious awareness and secondarily a lowering of inhibitory influences, it permits recollection of repressed, unpleasant experiences and their accompanying emotions. Abreaction may therefore be encouraged by inducing hypnosis.

The arguments for and against the use of hypnosis as a therapeutic maneuver have continued unabated since the days of Mesmer. The principal case of the opponents is that although there does appear to be a hypnotic state, its development, maintenance, and disappearance are inexplicable in terms of observable nervous system activity. The protagonists claim that it does no harm and that often it is beneficial in eliminating a discomfort, for example that of dental extraction or painful instrumentations.

Insofar as it can be said that any form of treatment which makes for more comfort at minimal risk has to be permitted, an open mind has to be kept about the therapeutic use of hypnosis.

ADVICE. Frequently, a point is reached in the first interview when advice is sought about some immediately pressing matter. "Do you think I should move? I find it difficult to take care of my house because I have too many rooms." The question may be a loaded one intended to trap the therapist into condoning some activity which is counter to the advice or interests of some other person.

For this reason, it is of the highest importance to avoid a yes or no answer which might either condone or antagonize. This is done by reflecting back to the decision-making by some comment such as, "I wonder why you feel incapable of making that decision." Even a question which is put at the social level has undertones significant to the therapeutic relationship.

The therapist may fear that being noncommital will frustrate, and this may be so, but it will lead to less difficulties in the long run than converting the visits into a game in which attempts are made to get desired answers and the therapist offers them.

VENTILATION. Opportunity to ventilate in an emotionally neutral and permissive atmosphere convinces that all can be told without fear of disturbing the listener, who is following meticulously, but nonjudgmentally. The sick person is seething with feelings of guilt, hostility, or other nonbenign sentiments. Failure to obtain from the helper a negative reaction, enhances the subject's feelings of security about both himself and his auditor. His own bad feelings cannot be so very bad if they cause no remonstrance, not even the lifting of an eyebrow.

The time permitted to allow self-expression at a rate compatible with emotional tolerance indicates an attempt to understand rather than merely to pry. Interventions in the form of open-ended questions invite expansion upon what the examiner would like to hear. The estimate of the importance of what is being said is left to the patient. Ventilation and its therapeutic value can be an important aspect of improvements of a dramatic nature after an initial interview.

CLARIFICATION. Except for hypnosis, any one or more of the foregoing is used almost unwittingly by the therapist in his daily contacts with patients. A technique about which he should be more aware, because he could use it to good advantage, especially when he feels that he is being pressured to make a decision which he is unwilling to offer, is clarification. Counseling as opposed— if indeed, it can be—to psychotherapy is being offered now by so many professionals who work directly with people that a word about its pitfalls is in order here. Counseling of course, implies giving advice. While a physician is certainly within his clinical rights in giving advice regarding such matters as medication and dietary restrictions, one may question if therapists should ever give advice regarding one's way of life and behavior. There are many reasons for this, ranging from avoiding delusions of omnipotence to avoiding blame for advice going wrong.

It is urged that one not go beyond clarification, and never be an umpire or a judge when told, "I know this is my problem: should I do this, or that?" The most to be done in that situation is to expose the issue and let the client work out for himself what might be the outcome. Help will be given in guiding the lines of thought and in hinting at possible new ones by suitable questions. This will be a kind of prodding to help push aside those prejudices and other emotional blocks which obscure the real difficulties and thereby prevent their examination. There are certainly many exceptions where the circumstances may make problem-solving irrelevant and dependency may at times be encouraged.

One would hope that individual obscurities might become rearrangeable for ease in resolution. The desirable activity is to restate as simply and clearly as possible the posed itemized problems, but with a question mark. Even this may be considered, under certain circumstances, as too active an intervention, in that the clarifying is then being done by others. It might be more enlightening if encouragement were given by a request: "Would you please repeat that?" with or without, "I don't quite following your meaning." An intervention that may seem more blunt and yet is paradoxically more indirect is the comment, "You seem to have a need to confuse yourself in this matter." While trying to prove the speaker wrong, the patient may surprise himself by a new-found clarity in such a restatement of his anxieties.

Exclamations such as "really," "well," "perhaps," "it could be so," and "naturally" are statements used in nearly all psychotherapeutic procedures. Several interesting items of activity are mentioned by Dollard and Miller (1950). By noticing certain things and neglecting others, responses are strengthened. The therapist's attention is a strong reward. "Uhuh" may be used in some sentences and not in others. "Mmmhmm" may be used similarly. Repeating in a questioning manner something said which is contradictory to something else—"But you can be more independent now"—is used to encourage the patient away from dependency.

Abreaction is a form of emotional release expressed with a greater or lesser degree of control appropriate to the setting and circumstances. If there is weeping to relieve intense sorrow, this is generally uninhibited. If intense anger is evoked, this may be seen in the form of muscular and vascular and other responses to autonomic impulses; a cigarette may be stubbed violently, or a pipestem broken, but overt violence is rarely exhibited.

Any feeling or mixture of feelings which floods the consciousness and is expressed as freely and as comfortably as is invited by the rapport is an abreaction and has a potential for a corrective emotional experience. When the emotional storm has subsided, the opportunity should be taken to discuss, in more tempered circumstances, the feelings which have been demonstrated and the object which has stimulated them and against which they are directed.

It might be mentioned in passing that the first abreactive experience is not necessarily a cure. One good bout of weeping or one clear manifestation of somewhat suppressed but nevertheless intense anger is rarely that effective. The exciting stresses and consequent feelings may have to be mentally lived through at repeated intervals to allow their impact to diminish. Such experience encourages, as it were, a graduated decompression of chronic tension and a consequent amelioration of bodily discomfort.

INTERPRETATION. By this is meant the explanation of a significance which has not yet been appreciated between a past event and the patient's emotional reaction to it. This significance may be clear to the therapist from a combination of what has already been revealed and what experience with other similar cases has taught him, or it may be that the patient has told everything but has not himself succeed in making the linkage.

An interpretation, however psychodynamically accurate, usually only mystifies when thrust at a person. Generally, it is a more gratifying maneuver which has been marked by the therapist as nuclear in the development of the disability. Emotions which were aroused by the happening have become mingled and unclear or even completely forgotten. Repeated recounting of the story from all possible angles is encouraged in the hope that the actual emotions that occurred with, and in reaction to, the event will be both recalled and assigned to it. A leading question here and there may be appropriate if the patient persistently dodges the issue, but one should beware not to be too hasty lest there be a recurrence of the anxiety which the emotionally turbulent incident had originally engendered. Most often, it is found that given forbearance, he either will find the interpretation himself or quite clearly show that he is eager and ready to receive it.

Estimation of progress must not be dependent upon only what he feels. He may say he is indeed "feeling better" and may even look to be so, but a true reflection of his progress is to be found in a change in his ability to manage relationships with others.

This epitomizes the ultimate of psychotherapy. The sick person wants relief from symptoms; the therapist's first task is to make him understand that these arise from real and fantasized problems he has with people both in the present and in memories of his past. He has been invited to try to solve, with the guidance of the therapist, at least the more accessible of these. Evidence of success will be seen in a more tolerant and considerate way of dealing with others, arising from an increase in self-esteem and confidence; he will become more giving and less self-conscious, more able to receive without guilt, and more decisive without being impetuous. Besides which, he will have fewer symptoms.

This is a much more modest goal than the alteration in personality, achievement of emotional maturity, or dissolution of repression. It is more realistic since even a limited problem-solving venture is not accepted by the elderly in large numbers. One may find interpretation to be a tool used infrequently with the more sophisticated elderly person.

Toward the end of the first interview, the therapist should have some inkling as to the interest of the patient in returning. If this is at all evident, he should discuss the contract—the arrangement of appointments, fees, conditions to be met in regard to failures to meet appointments and whatever else is thought necessary to consolidate as far as possible the "rituals" of psychotherapy. There may be a need to imply that help is indeed indicated and is available, but care must be taken to avoid assurance of improvement or cure. If the patient vacillates about returning, the response will depend upon how sick he is judged to be. If he is clearly suicidal or homicidal, the question of admission to the hospital will have to be discussed both with him and with his next of kin—preferably with his consent, but not necessarily so in such a potentially dangerous situation.

If, as is much more often the case, he is able to go about his affairs although in a less than effective way, the therapist must avoid any suspicion of coercing or persuading him to return, above all, by any suggestion that might be misunderstood as some sort of threat. Even if the therapist has written off the possibility that the patient will return to him, it is not wise to say more than "I cannot tell if you will get worse without treatment, but I believe you will more likely get to understand and find solutions to your problems with the help of someone who can be objective about your difficulties." This will leave a clean and uncluttered field for a fresh start.

The parting should be on a note of willingness to reconsider at any time another call for help regardless of the termination of this first meeting or series of meetings: and also always on a note of cautious optimism. It is possible that one may believe he can make no change in a patient with a severe character disorder, and one may feel it only honest to refuse to enter into any therapeutic contract with him. But it would be kinder to leave the implication that this is a weakness in one's own skill rather than a difficulty inherent in the disorder and to suggest that there may be others who can offer help in a similar or different way.

Summary

It is possible in a communicating relationship to get a fair idea of what is really troublesome, what short-term and what long-term events have led up to the situation, how much can be done, and how accepting an offer to help.

All this can be evoked with a minimum of open-ended, neutrally-toned and nonprovocative questions designed to elicit the story in a spiral interlocking of events. Asking a series of direct questions will certainly give a straight-line, compartmentalized history with an emphasis on events: The history, spontaneously related, usually puts the greater emphasis on the feelings which have been associated with the events. This is not only informative for the therapist, but, to a greater or lesser degree, both revelatory and cathartic.

It is not proposed to outline here, as in the usual textbook type of example page, a list of spheres of interest for the therapist, such as school and work histories, sexual development, marital history, and the like. Of more significance to therapy is that anything of importance in any such sphere will eventually come to light if the listener is manifestly interested and is sufficiently aware of dynamic processes to seek parallels in the different areas of the life chosen for discussion. If he is obviously avoiding talk about his work, this should be a sufficient clue to the therapist to edge some inquiry gently into that direction.

The first interview is usually structured by the often unspoken understanding that the complaints will be stated. This might proceed to a history of the origins of these and even to some account of personal and family history with the nondirective guidance of the therapist. A time arrives, sooner or later, when there is a halt in the flow. Then explicitly, or implicitly, questions are likely to follow. "What am I supposed to do now?" He is trying to convey that this is all he thinks that needs to be told; possibly even that this is all he can remember as having even the remotest connection with the troubles which have brought him to seek help.

CONFRONTATION PROBLEM-SOLVING PSYCHOTHERAPY

The theoretic, scientific frame of reference of all varieties of psychotherapy remains open to question. This holds true for orthodox psychoanalysis through all its modifications and heresies. Based on a theory on the development of a problem-solving attitude or conditioned reaction of compliance with or without critical appraisal and evaluation, a system is offered of a therapeutic approach in which it is expected that the patient will soon come to understand his own role. It is hoped that he will learn that this is not a passive one; that he is there not only to be helped; he is also there to be shown how he can help himself. The therapist preferably does not see himself as a donor of health. He is a guide who is able to lead into an understanding of how one can go about improving oneself. This is done by showing that emotional troubles come from a conditioned inability to solve everyday problems of living. This inability is a repetitive pattern going back to a time when either a person became accustomed to having problems solved for him whenever the need arose, or was content with only partial solutions which gave at least temporary results. This is introduced to him not by words and explanations, but by the technical process of this therapeutic plan which is intended to make him see that there are problems to be solved, and that he must help solve them himself, and this applies not only to current problems, but even to those of the past, the unsatisfactory solutions of which have set the pattern for his subsequent bedevilled course of existence. Experience with colleagues who have graduated from a variety of training programs indicates that one can teach theory, but so far there is no way in which to teach practice.

One is generally motivated to seek psychotherapeutic help by two conflicting wishes or desires. A client may seek help from a magical healer to reinforce strivings against impulses threatening danger and to bring about restoration to health. In its deepest sense, this would mean the gratification of all impulses, hopes, desires, and expectations. Possibly, what the sick person is seeking is the reestablishment of that state in which his basic defenses are no longer threatened. Masserman described these as the "Ur defenses." They are, in paraphrase:

(1) Denial of danger and death maintains the delusion of invulnerability and immortality.

(2) The creation of God in the image of man assures the external presence of an all-controlling and protective force which can be evoked by prayer and worship and gifts to come to man's aid in time of need.

(3) A belief in an instinctive philanthropy and benevolence means that in the last resort there must always be human help.

Many hopes, expectations, and desires are prevented from fulfillment, not because of any real barrier, but rather because of attitudes and feelings about these wishes, needs, and desires. At one time, they were related realistically to the situation in childhood. However, they no longer have positive adaptive value in the current and future life. These currently nonadaptive patterns of behavior were initiated during the development of the infantile neuroses and reinforced throughout life. The individual develops methods for dealing with his environment and with objects of importance in the world: namely, with significant individuals with whom he comes in close contact—his mother, father, and siblings. The breakdown in psychological balance occurs because the methods of dealing habitually with internal and external stimuli, developed throughout life, prove to be an insufficiently adequate method for dealing with the stresses of an adult world during the years of decline.

The following maneuver was devised and used with the hope that this technique would enhance the work of psychotherapy. Several methods of wording statements were developed which sought to clarify the conflicts and issues. One method was to use an authoritative statement directing control of certain drives, impulses, or desires. This was then followed by the question: "What do you think and feel about what I told you?" The use of a direct statement by the therapist has value in that it creates a situation wherein the person can feel that if his own ability to control the undesirable impulse or to function independently is impaired, then such control will emanate from outside sources. Controlling through methods which reestablish the authoritarian parent-child relationship is generally frowned upon or may be considered, at best, a form of supportive psychotherapy intended to strengthen *superego* action against forbidden, but self-destructive, drives. It reassures, however, that one's controls will be strengthened further by an external control, and thus relieves acute panic states and anxiety. Such authoritarian control tends to intensify the tendency to repeat a behavior pattern previously executed without question as to its significance. When, however, the statement is associated with insistence that one explore thoughts, feelings, and the necessity or desirability of complying, by the question, "What do you think and feel about what I told you?", a desire to test the significance of controls and to evaluate these further on a realistic basis is created. The therapist has fostered reality testing in contradistinction to fostering dependence. The use of the statement may also strengthen the feelings of hopeful recovery and restoration to health. Since a great deal of faith in the ability to recover has been lost, the promise of health increases the capacity to deal with anxieties and to be aware of the conflicts creating his anxiety. Then, freed from anxiety, one can construct more wholesome and more realistic adaptations. The struggle of primitive impulses, seeking expression against the internalized controls becomes partially transferred to a conflict between those impulses and an external, prohibiting parental figure and leads to an awareness of the attitudes toward such impulses in the sociocultural milieu. Similar authoritarian maneuvers are used to support symptoms which represent acceptable impulses, prohibitions, or coping activity. In each instance, the meaning of the statement is subjected to exploration by the question, "What do you think and feel about what I told you?"

The special activity called the "Confrontation Problem-Solving Technique" was founded in the context of a psychoanalytically oriented, therapeutic process. Its value became quickly apparent as the repetitive stimulus encouraged exploration of a conflict selected by the therapist as being the most immediately disabling. In some individuals, as is generally accepted, it is neither possible nor desirable to do more than restore emotional ease by encouraging repression of a conflict which is threatening to break through in some uncomfortable disguise. Here it was found that a suitable statement of confrontation could be derived from the conscious expression of this threat. The statement, followed by the question, or the latter only, used repetitively as indicated, can produce effective repression and relief from symptoms.

The nature of the statement varies with the goals of therapy, the personality structure, or the nature of what is currently the most disturbing conflict. Usually it is a conflict about which the person is conscious or which is operating at a preconscious level: the goal may be insight and some increase in personality flexibility or simply an alleviation of symptoms by reestablishing an equilibrium previously present, usually by the therapist encouraging repression.

In the course of therapy, the statement of confrontation needs to be repeated from time to time, and its subsequent question should be repeated much more often, in the form of "What do you think and feel about what I told you?"

The question may be asked when material directly related to the statement is being expressed, or when the material is clearly derivative of, or substitutive for, a reaction to the statement. Also, the question can often usefully be reintroduced during long, anxiety-provoking (for the therapist) silences as an alternative to, or as a follow-up after some comment to the effect that "You seem to be having trouble telling me what your thoughts are now."

The statement of confrontation can be determined by the immediate, unsatisfactorily resolved problem and concomitant conflict.

It may be, therefore:

(1) a prohibitive statement, e.g. or "I want you to stop your alcoholic habits at once."
(2) a permissive statement, e.g. "It would be better if you rid yourself of your husband."
(3) an adaptive statement involving mature value orientations: "I want you to continue at work regardless of your employer's attitude."

It is of the utmost importance that whenever the confronting statement is made, it be followed with question, "What do you think and feel about what I told you?"

In formulating the wording of the confrontation statement, the therapist might, depending on the circumstances:

(1) state very clearly a problem which is crucial, but is not at all, or only vaguely, recognized;
(2) present in an exaggerated or paradoxical manner an actual solution to the problem in order to illuminate possible action;
(3) offer in an exaggerated statement what the end results of continued maladaptive activity might be, as a stimulus toward discontinuing such behavior.

The repetitive statement concerning the conflict or the suggested solution should make it evident that the current situation is untenable and unacceptable and that a real solution can be found by continuous searching. It is also as if the therapist's subsequent repetition of the question acts as a continuous pressure to force the acceptance of a need to explore and solve the unearthed problem.

The confrontation technic can be looked upon as stimulating certain percepts. The percepts are then subjected to a continuous critical reappraisal by the question: "What do you think and feel about what I told you?" The confrontation technic therefore, may help fill the need for finding a way to bring about a correction of incorrect perceptions. There is a tendency for incorrect perceptions not to be corrected on the basis of new experiences because the anxiety associated with the new experiences, or a person's chronic statement of anxiety tends to create an avoidance reaction to any appropriate reevaluation of an incorrect perception. The importance of perception and perceptual errors in the confrontation technic is attested to by the frequency of times the patient *does not perceive* what he has been told.

The immediate reply to the question on its first presentation depends to a large extent upon the attitude of transference and the immediate feelings. There may be a complete silence, followed by a comment which suggests that the statement has not (as has been mentioned above) even been heard; or a response tinged with hostility: "That's just exactly what I've been wanting to do: I don't need you to tell me!" "How can you say such a terrible thing—I don't want my husband to die!"; or a quick demonstration of a desire to comply. But whatever the response, mixed feelings will be obvious: surprise, of course, mingled with varying degrees of anxiety, fear, impatience, and— hopefully—curiosity. If an insight has been illuminated, there will also be pain. "You know I want my husband to live" may well be accompanied with a sudden, conscious realization that death wishes have indeed existed—and shame and guilt are added to the emotional mixture. But the response most hoped for is curiosity.

The confronting statement followed by the question is intended to reveal the current problem; that it is up to the person to solve it, but with the help of the therapist; for the latter asks, "What do *you* think and feel about what *I* told you?"

In headlong flight from reality, controls, and object relations, the patient finds himself confronted by the therapist in such a way that his line of retreat is cut off. If he wishes to evade reality now, he has to think about why. But thinking about reasons for evading reality requires differentiating among reasons, evaluating them, and choosing how to behave. The crumbling controls are reinforced. Anxiety is reduced. Also, one is invited to explore one's problems with the help and support of someone who has obviously done his part in bridging the communication barrier.

During the treatment, the process of developing self-assurance through mastery and achievement is not inhibited by fear of punishment, shame, failure, or loss of love because of the non-condemning nature of the relationship and the encouragement to seek a solution suggested by the repetitive question.

The more the therapist wishes to achieve by uncovering and by producing a corrective emotional experience, the more important it is to focus the confronting statement upon the core problem. That statement will change, therefore, as it outlives its usefulness, and it becomes necessary to devise a new one, appropriate to each still unresolved problem.

The suggestion offered here (to use a statement followed by the request that the patient himself explore its significance) constitutes a relatively constant psychotherapeutic technique. It is suggested that the statement-question as a stimulus to problem-solving (confrontation technic) focuses acute attention on fixed attitudes, beliefs, and maladaptive processes. These have, to a large degree, become automatic routines for dealing with life experiences, based essentially on old fears of loss of love, or punishment by parents or parental figures. In response to the statement-question, the patient many times experiences emotional reactions similar to those previously evoked by circumstances with parents and parent surrogates. However, the question, directed at encouraging him to express his thoughts or feelings about the statement, leads to a reexploration of these past experiences and of their significance for his present life. It also reveals the nature of the treatment as a means of exploring the reaction to significant figures in the present. It is suggested that the technic described has some specific possibilities as a research tool in dealing with psychotherapeutic methods. By studying one particular statement and the responses to it through time, one might discover some possibly significant alterations in the patterning of psychodynamic material. The reactions to one particular statement, over the period of treatment, may be classified as variables to a fixed stimulus. The changing of the responses to such a fixed stimulus may enable one to measure change in the patient through time.

Management of the Patient with Cancerophobia

Patients seek examinations for reasons other than the presence of illness requiring medical help. A frequent reason is the feeling that physical illness exists when in fact it does not. Less involved in the concern over cancer than the severely ill, obsessive-compulsive person is the one with a mildly exaggerated concern over physical well-being. He may ask that his stomach be examined or complain of discomfort in some part of the body and may incidentally point out that some member of the family died of cancer. The obvious conclusion, that he is seeking reassurance, may be further verified by other remarks during the visit.

If an individual recently had a complete examination, a thorough examination of the organ which is the basis for the complaint is desirable. For instance, if the complaints are coughing and chest pain, the heart and lungs should be examined. The examination should be followed by a positive statement: "It seems the recent death (or other circumstances) created some concern about cancer. I wish to tell you definitely I find no evidence of cancer. Your symptoms reflect your concern about the problem. You know I have an appointment to see you for your yearly physical examination."

If seen for the first time, with a mildly exaggerated concern over his health he should first receive a complete physical examination. He should then receive the explanations to be described for the person with obsessive preoccupation with illness.

There are many who seek examinations because of an obsessive preoccupation with the possibility of having a dread disease. In recent years, cancerophobia has replaced syphilophobia as a frequent obsessive preoccupation. When seen for the first time, the person with cancerophobia should receive a thorough investigation by history-taking, physical examination and laboratory studies. When told the results of the examination, and it is fairly definite that cancer is not a cause for concern, it is best to reassure him in a positive manner: "I have examined you and find no evidence of any disease. I specifically wish to tell you that my examination and the tests show absolutely no evidence of cancer." A continued search for the explanation of further complaints with each visit is usually not in his best interest and he is given the explanation that the yearly physical examination is usually sufficient. When the compulsive insistence requires it, examination of an organ or part of the body may be desirable. Subsequent visits are best managed by emphasizing his difficulty in accepting what he is told in a statement such as the one below. The statement, however, should be preceded by careful hearing of the complaints and symptoms: "You seem to have a good deal of doubt about my judgment. You seem to feel I should tell you again that I haven't found cancer. Since I've already told you so, you must have doubts about trusting my conclusion. I wonder why?"

Invariably the patient will feel that the doctor feels insulted and will try to reassure him. When he seeks reassurance again, the appropriate response is a shrug of the shoulders and a reiteration of the fact that he was already told cancer doesn't exist. "I wonder why you feel it is necessary for me to tell you again." Reexaminations and repeated reassurances often fit into his need to doubt that the original examination was not complete enough or that the truth was withheld.

The somatic delusion of having cancer may be the central core of the disability in a person seemingly well organized in most areas of personality functioning. The transition from a severe obsessive-compulsive neurosis to that of a psychotic distubance is not sharply defined. I cannot agree with Branch (1952) who believes such patients are not reluctant to accept psychiatric help if the suggestion is made tactfully by the examining physiican. He writes:

> These are difficult cases to handle and treatment from any point of view is long and often disappointing. The fear of cancer amounts to a nuclear psychosis, a real delusion, and arises from a tremendous guilt reaction which demands as punishment the 'rotting away' of the individual. These patients will sometimes admit that

no amount of physical examination or reassurance completely dispels their conviction that cancer is lurking somewhere.

Repeated examinations and reassurance are often interpreted as evidence that the examiner is uncertain or is covering up the true facts. Psychiatric referral is desirable, although one must admit that, on the whole, the psychiatrist has not been too successful if fixed somatic delusions exist. If referral is refused, the following techniques may represent the best approach to treatment:

(1) Seek more information about the patient's life. Listen, rather than spending time in repeated examinations.

(2) Limit investigation after the initial complete physicial examination to the part about whch there is a complaint; do this only when the anxiety seems to be unalleviated without such an examination.

(3) Confront the patient with his inability to accept the information given him: "Apparently, you feel you can't trust my examination and my judgment about you. I wonder why? Why do you insist on believing you have cancer?"

This technique avoids fortification of the delusional thinking. It makes it quite evident that the physician does not accept a physical basis for the complaints. Further, the questions suggest that exploration into life's situations and the need to believe something which is not so, is desirable. It is true that the patient may not be satisfied with such an approach and may seek other medical help. However, one can have the satisfaction of knowing that no harm has been done. A special confrontation technic described by the author has been successful in treatment of patients with somatic delusions. Electroshock treatment may sometimes bring about a remission in the symptoms and lobotomy may be considered as a last resort.

Management of the Patient with Cancer

What to tell the patient who has cancer has been of increasing interest to the medical profession as the focus in practice moved from the concept of treating the disease to treating the person. There has likewise been considerable emphasis placed on the education of the public as to the cause and prevention of illness, with the professionals directing attention to symptoms, prognosis, and treatment, but also warning against the possibility of the dread malady if careful inspection of the body is not carried out at frequent intervals.

Renneker (1952) aptly expressed the difficulty:

> Each doctor tends to work out a method according to his own feelings or lack of feelings about the problem. We believe that this leads to hit-and-miss methods which often cause unnecessary emotional trauma to the patient. The common denominators in these miscellaneous approaches revolve around techniques of grave concealment or giving misleading partial information accompanied by an attempt at reassurance.

The *humanly factural approach* to telling the patient about cancer is one which I feel is not generally desirable. This approach described by Renneker is probably satisfactory for the person who finds denial difficult, but is able to develop considerable hope and faith, especially when the transferential relationship to the physician encourages this. When using the humanly factual approach, the physician, having told the patient that cancer is the diagnosis, acquaints him with the encouraging details of prognosis and treatment. The necessary therapeutic steps of biopsy, mastectomy, or radiation, and their importance are explained. The suggestion to pay attention to the status of the emotional health and "not allow the patient to build up and retain unnecessary fears and feelings of inevitable death" (Renneker, 1952), is not followed by any information as to how this be done.

The immediate presurgical management must be related to the nature of the surgery to be performed. The severely deforming surgical procedures about the head and neck should enlist all possible psychological helps. An explanation of the disease and the facts pertinent to it, even though this has an immediately depressing effect, will serve to mitigate the anxieties. From a moral point of view the patient is entitled to be informed of the facts of his case, and they should not be withheld unless there is clear-cut evidence that knowledge of the truth will be detrimental. The amount of factual information to be imparted is an individual question. Kindness, understanding and personal interest soften the bitterest facts.

A brief discussion of the postoperative period, length of time of hospitalization and the period of rehabilitation at home will prepare the person for the entire experience. A majority, appropriately prepared, go on to accept surgery; some go hysterically from one doctor to another seeking a solution acceptable to them; some avoid surgery only to return when the prognosis has been worsed; and finally, some, in the full knowledge of the prognosis, go on with equanimity (aided by alcohol and narcotics), feeling they have no reason to make a struggle against such a deadly enemy.

Being untruthful is never (or perhaps hardly ever) justifiable, although a family member who feels he knows best may suggest deception. A diagnosis other than a truthful one should be avoided if possible, even if it is suggested by the family. (The discovery of the deception creates a lack of truth which precludes the possibility of frank discussions about illness and dying.) "distortion of reality for the sake of soporific support violates the relationship between doctor and patient fully as much as does a blunt confrontation with the unmitigated facts" (Weisman, 1962). Too often the dishonesty is associated with a certain behavior on the part of the family and treatment procedures which only an imbecile would fail to recognize. I find it difficult to comprehend how a physician can tell a patient with cancer that he is suffering from neuritis and at the same time refer him for x-ray therapy during which he spends many hours talking to others with cancer. One could hardly fail to grasp the significance of his treatment except through massive denial.

By following the procedure to be described, one can be truthful at all times, although the truth is an incomplete account of the facts.

The first evidence of cancer may be disclosed at the time of an examination of a routine nature. The following is set forth as a series of steps which may be used as a guide to a *psychotherapeutic communication*. I wish to emphasize that there can be no fixed rule: "There can only be a physician with a heart"

(Litin *et al.*, 1960). Truth will be the essence of the approach suggested. The truth will be qualified by limiting information so that a careful understanding of the individuals needs will direct the guidelines. If the patient is to be examined by others—for example, if an internist intends to have a surgeon see him and if pathological studies are to be done—it is wise not to make a definitive diagnosis at this point, since there is a possibility that the first clinical impression may not be completely correct.

After the examination has disclosed pathology indicating the presence of a tumor the patient is told, "I have found a tumor (or 'something wrong'). I wish to have you examined by Dr. Z and have tests made." If accepted without question there need be no further information given. But if he then asks, "What kind of tumor? Is it a cancer, Doctor?" the reply might best be, "I wonder why you should expect the unpleasant. I don't know as yet. Let us both wait until we have more information." When information has come from the laboratory, or an affirming diagnostic conclusion has been reached, the person must be prepared for a surgical or other treatment procedure, and is told, "You have a growth (or tumor) requiring surgery. The surgery may require the removal of (whatever organ is involved)." If accepted without question, there need be no elaboration. One can assume that denial of illness as a defense is being established. When the patient seeks additional information, such as "If you have to remove the breast, I have cancer, don't I?" I believe that this question may frequently be based on a desire to fortify a need for denial which is as yet not fully established. The question is best answered by, "I wonder why you have to believe the unpleasant." If there is a strong need for denial of illness there may be a fortification of the defense and acceptance will take place without further questioning. The patient may seek a more definitive answer at this time and may recognize the physician's stalling tactics. One can remain discreet and yet honest in one's reply: "It must be obvious to you that we suspect the tumor is malignant, but there can never be an absolute answer. The surgery and pathology studies will help determine the nature of the growth."

There are those who seek treatment for symptoms of relatively recent origin, but in whom cancer may be suspected. The person with a somewhat persistent cough or a change in bowel function may induce the physician to require further diagnostic investigation. The discussion of a differential diagnosis including the possibility of malignancy is not wise. If asked for the reason for further tests, the doctor might indicate that he is obligated to reasonable thoroughness in seeking for the meaning of the symptoms. If the patient is hesitant about becoming involved in extensive investigation, the physician may be positive and firm in saying, "It is important for you that this be done. Inflammations and other conditions, curable when treated early, may be causing your symptoms." The patient may then ask, "Do you suspect cancer?" The answer might be "I wonder why you have to suspect the unpleasant. There are many conditions of minor significance that could cause the same symptoms." If the patient persists with "Doctor, I know you wouldn't have to go through these tests if you weren't suspicious of cancer," the response might be, "It is true that I have to consider such a possibility, but the probabilities are against such a diagnosis," or, "It is one possibility among others."

The person who has recognized the doctor's tactics and who wishes to have more information may be resigning himself to helpless, discouraged hopelessness about the future. It is important never to present a hopeless picture. The degree to which help and encouragement can be given is dependent to some extent on the prognosis for the cancer from which he is suffering. The dermatologist frequently tells his patient that cancer is present because he can be encouraging and helpful to the point of being quite assured about an excellent outcome. It is obvious that it might be particularly useful, especially if the prognosis is good, to point out the positive, helpful potential that exists in the surgery and the treatment. There need be no discussion of the details of surgery, X-rays, glands, etc. The query, "But, Doctor, I have cancer?" is best responded to by a question, "Yes, but I wonder why you have to see it as so hopeless a condition? I have known many patients who have recovered from cancer." Emphasis on what will be done to help must highlight any further discussion.

After surgery has been done, it is best to postpone any discussion until the patient is reasonably comfortable. If the patient is satisfied with previous discussions and complete clarification seems unnecessary, the establishment of an atmosphere of treatment, encouragement, and hope as stimulated by the behavior and attitude of the physician may be all that is necessary. The person who has accepted an incomplete answer may continue to fortify denial of illness, and, unless otherwise indicated, the diagnosis of tumor or growth does not require further elaboration. The person who cannot accept an indefinite answer may now seek to establish a definitive diagnosis. "What did you find, Doctor?" He may respond "A tumor was found in your breast and the breast was removed." She may not seek other information and may fortify the denial of the seriousness of the pathology. If she seeks a more direct answer with "But, Doctor, was it a cancer?" the answers and maneuvers best for the postsurgical patient are, "Yes, you have a cancer," followed by an elaboration of all encouraging aspects of prognosis and treatment which are appropriate to the nature of the cancer and to the patient's overall condition.

As indicated previously the basic or primary defenses, important to the maintenance of mental well-being, are significant for the cancer patient and the dying patient. Essentially, these defenses are (1) a belief in one's own invulnerability. We are able to be objective about death when it is seen as impersonal. Intrapersonal death is something we cannot comprehend. (2) The belief in an omnipotent helper or the inherent need to feel that some omnipotent force is available to protect us from harm and danger may be evident. (3) The belief in the helpfulness of one's fellowman is important. All of these defenses have been fortified and strengthened in the person who responds to the postsurgical period with a degree of well-being not anticipated by the seriousness of the illness. The basic defenses strengthen the positive feelings for the physician. To him is transferred the expectation of help, care, interest and affection that was originally felt for important persons in the past—especially the parents. Much of the comfort throughout the trying days ahead will be determined by how the interpersonal patient-physician relationship is managed.

In the months following surgery, the individual who may have accepted incomplete information about the illness may, for one of a number of reasons, reopen the question of diagnosis: "What's wrong with me? Do I have cancer?" One should not overlook the possibility that he or she wishes encouragement for a denial of illness. The responses should deal with the resistance to accepting what was an acceptable solution to anxiety. "Apparently, you don't feel you can accept what I told you." The reason for the patient asking the question will then be clarified. If his need is to strengthen denial there will be no questions, or a response such as, "What you told me is good enough for me." If the patient is not satisfied with the answer, he will seek a more specific one: "Tell me, do I or don't I have cancer?" The response might then be, "If I tell you that you have cancer you may believe nothing can be done. Yet, in honesty, I must tell you that our tests and examination confirm such a diagnosis." This type of response might be followed by all the encouragement and hopeful statements that are warranted. An elaboration of the treatment available, and possibly the statement, " I know many who have been cured of cancer," may supply the necessary stimulus for a hopeful, rather than hopeless, view of the future. The above interpersonal interchange does not preclude frank discussions in which identity, dignity, self-respect, and worth are maintained.

Treatment methods directed at externalizing the interests and creating new sources of gratification can be broadly applied. In management of patients who may vary considerably in their needs, one can only individualize treatment accordingly. The terminal individual is obviously an entirely different problem than the patient operated upon disabled to some degree by the physical changes, but with a long life expectancy. The person with cervical carcinoma discovered early and with a hopefully complete cure with no significant physical disability is not beset by the problems of one who is physially mutilated and has limited functions. For cervical carcinoma, postoperative care may require nothing more than judicious management and an air of hopeful, nonconcerned interest. The avoidance of creating an atmosphere that suggests nothing further can be done is all that may be required.

For the functionally disabled, the limitations of activity enforced must be realistically appraised. Planning of treatment activities must show a common sense awareness of the personality, social status and interests, economic situation, work interests, and possibly, above all, the family structure. An activity therapy program may be instituted in the hospital and fostered, directed and encouraged by the treating physician. Some activities which may be crucial for the patient's total well-being and social functioning follow:

1) intellectual achievements and interests which are gratifying
2) developing social skills and activities
3) promoting and expanding sports interests
4) source-finding skills for expansion of and participation in new recreations
5) achieving skills and promoting interests in fine arts, music, dance, dramatics, writing and crafts
6) demonstrating the possibilities in home economics skills through gratification in knowledge and achievements in cooking, entertaining, sewing, and other homemaking skills.
7) in the case of children and youngsters, helping to arrange for continuation of education with school authorities.

Where resources enable him to seek out and participate in enjoyable and gratifying life experiences there need be no attempt to convert a treat for the person into a treatment. For those who need the type of structured activity outlined above, more information is required about motivation, level of aspiration, tolerance for frustration and many other psychophysical correlates which will play important roles in the reaction to illness.

Treatment of the dependency problems varies with whether the dependency needs are being expressed in a person who has previously maintained a reasonably mature and constructive attitude toward problems in living under stress, or if immature, infantile insatiable demanding was characteristic throughout his life. If the former is true, then a supportive sympathetic acceptance of the dependency is reasonable until there is evidence of using the position of dependency for gratification when it is no longer warranted.

When the person with insatiable dependency needs and immaturity of character becomes ill, the problem is compounded. A vicious cycle may develop as he makes more demands than the personnel in the hospital feel are necessary. As the personnel fails to respond to the demands, anxiety and anger mount and the demands are increased. The personnel respond to the increased demands with increased resentment and intentional neglect which in turn leads to an irritable, and even more intractable patient. The end result of the cycle is a need to prove that the demands were justified by developing more symptoms and greater disability.

The management should include a series of steps which will lessen demanding and decrease the disability. I believe the following management will be fairly successful: a firm, sympathetic attitude with passive listening and selective attention to the positive statements. When the demanding is associated with complaints of improper care, the response of the therapist should be one which could lead to a realistic evaluation of the demanding attitude. "Apparently you feel I am not being sufficiently concerned with your care," or "you feel I am inconsiderate of your needs," "do not have enough sympathy for your problems," and so on. Such a response will lead to exploration of the patient's demanding nature: expressions of hostility over improper care which have a realistic base; an uncovering to the patient of the meaning of the therapist, and so on. The therapist's noncondemning attitude toward expressions of hostility, sympathetic listening to problems, and correction of well-grounded complaints will often decrease demanding nature considerably.

When such management fails, the use of a confrontation technic may be successful. The statement, "Stop believing you can get everything you want immediately," followed by the question, "What do you think or feel about what I told you?" used repetitively, may have saluatory effects. The therapist must be a passive noncondemning listener after making the comment. If resentment is aroused, he may respond by such interpretations as, "You apparently feel hurt about what I told you and feel that you are justified in your demands."

Medication should be ordered so that it is given in small doses very frequently, thus in anticipation of needs. Personnel should not be given the feeling the therapist is humoring a bad child, but that he is sincerely concerned with the health of the patient. Aspirin, one grain (.06 gram) every hour may be given for complaints of pain. Adequate sedation at night to make sleep possible and gratifying may be difficult to achieve. Avoid P.R.N. orders which are often given with resentment by the personnel, are based upon the demand, and creates the very clinical impasse which is to be avoided. Encouragement of discussions of life's situations tends to remove concern with the physical self and promotes awareness of the real problem. Comments such as, "You must have found that a painful experience," may make the patient aware of the source of the real discomfort.

> Far older than the precept, 'the truth, the whole truth, and nothing but the truth,' is another that originates within our profession that has always been a guide to the best physicians, and, if I venture a prophecy, will always remain so; so far as possible, 'do no harm.' You can do harm by the processes which are quaintly called "telling the truth" or "lying." In your relations with patients, you will inevitably do much harm, and this will be by no means confined to your strictly medical blunders. It will also arise from what you say and what you fail to say. But try to do as little harm as possible, not only in treatment with drugs, or with the knife, but also in treatment with words, with the expression of your sentiments and emotions. Try at all times to act upon the patient so as to modify his sentiments to his own advantage, and remember that, to this end, nothing is more effective than arousing in him the belief that you are concerned wholeheartedly and exclusively for his welfare (Meyer, 1953).

That one must individualize as much as possible in keeping with past performance in stressful experiences should also be clear. Current life situations must be appraised in terms of the family's needs. A person's need to find a new executive to take care of a business upon which his family depends for economic support might decrease the possibility that the physician can accept denial of illness as a reasonable solution. One might have to respond so as to consider the sentiments of the patient and the needs of his family: "I think you should know that your problem is sufficiently serious so that you should consider plans for your family."

REFERENCES

Alexander, F.: Two forms of regression and therapeutic implications. *Psychoanal Q, 25*:176, 1956.

Berger, Milton (Ed.): *Video Tape Technique in Psychiatric Training and Treatment.* New York, Brunner-Mazel, 1970.

Branch, C. H.: The psychiatric approach to patients with malignant disease. *Rocky Mt Med J, 49*:749, 1952.

Dollard, J., and Miller, N. E.: *Personality and Psychotherapy.* New York, McGraw-Hill, 1950.

Garner, H. H.: Obtaining medical histories by indirect questioning. *Chicago Med Sch Q, 9*:19-22, 1948.

Garner, H. H., Simon, A. J., Handelman, M. S.: Management of chronic dependency in outpatient clinics by a comprehensive medical-psychiatry service. *J Am Geriat Soc, 61*:623-631, 1958.

Garner, H. H.: A confrontation technique used in psychotherapy. *Am J Psychother, 13*:18-34, 1959.

Garner, H. H.: Psychiatric aspects of surgery. *Industr Med Surg, 28*:351-361, 1959.

Garner, H. H.: Treatment—Review of a medical concept. *J Am Geriat Soc, 9*:833-910, 1961.

Garner, H. H.: Passivity and activity in psychotherapy. *Arch Gen Psychiatry, 5*:411-417, 1961.

Garner, H. H.: Interventions in psychotherapy and the confrontation interview. *Am J Psychoanal, 22*:47-58, 1962.

Garner, H. H.: Management of the patient with cancerophobia and cancer. *Psychosomatics, 5*:147-152, 1964.

Garner, H. H.: Management of the patient with malignant disease. Roche Report, Frontiers of Psychiatry in Clinical Medicine. *1*:5-6, 1965.

Garner, H. H.: Psychotherapy for the nonspecialist. *Psychosomatics, 6*:32-39, 1965.

Garner, H. H.: Compliance and problem-solving psychotherapy. *Compr Psychiatry, 7*:21-30, 1966.

Garner, H. H.: Somatopsychic concepts. *Psychosomatics, 7*:329-337, 1966.

Garner, H. H.: *Psychosomatic Management of the Patient with Malignancy.* Springfield, Thomas, 1966.

Garner, H. H.: Chronic Disability and the Sick Role. *Ill Med J, 132*:293-298, 1967.

Garner, H. H.: The medical interview and comprehensive patient care. *Psychosomatics, 9*:191-196, 1968.

Garner, H. H.: *Psychotherapy: Confrontation Problem-Solving Technique.* St. Louis, Green, 1970.

Harrower, Molly (Ed.): *Medical and Psychological Teamwork in the Care of the Chronically Ill.* Springfield, Thomas, 1955.

Hollender, M.: *The Psychology of Medical Practice.* Philadelphia, Saunders, 1958.

Litin, E., Rynearson, E., and Hallenbeck, G.: Symposium—What shall we tell the cancer patient? *Proc Mayo Clin, 35*:239-257, 1960.

Masserman, J.: Faith and delusion, in psychotherapy, Ur-defenses of man. *Am J Psychiatry, 110*:324, 1952.

Masserman, J.: *Practice of Dynamic Psychiatry.* Philadelphia, Saunders, 1953.

Meyer, B. C.: Should the patient know the truth? *J Mt Sinai Hosp, 20*:344, 1953.

Meyerson, Abraham: Psychosomatic and somatopsychics. *Psychiat, 14*:665, 1940.

Otto, J. L.: Psychosomatic aspects of cancer. *Rocky Mt Med J,* 49-50, April, 1961.

Renneker, R., and Cutler, M.: Psychological problems of adjustment to cancer of the breast. *JAMA, 148*:833, 1952.

Weinstein, E. A., and Kahn, R. L.: Denial of illness. Springfield, Thomas, 1955.

Weisman, A.: *The Dying Patient* (Lecture Series). Desplaines, Forest Hospital Publ, *1*:16, 1962.

Chapter 4

PSYCHOLOGICAL AND PSYCHOSEXUAL

ASPECTS OF ILEOSTOMY

MANAGEMENT*

ROBERT BLAKE

T HE PSYCHOLOGICAL ADJUSTMENT of the individual who becomes an ileostomate is so intimate a part of the disease process which eventually leads to colectomy and ileostomy, and so important in the adjustment of the patient to his new mode of excretion and its undeniable effects on his interpersonal relationships, that any approach to the subject of the ileostomate cannot be effective or adequate unless these aspects are fully appreciated. Sexual function of the individual is so dependent on his psychological balance that is cannot be considered except in this context. It seems most suitable to present the situation as it applies to the stages through which the patient progresses to the final outcome. Therefore, a chronological account will permit the most productive description of these facets of ileostomy care.

---

* Editors' Note: This chapter is presented as an example of the psychological and rehabilitative concerns of one specific type of cancer. There are many other examples which could have been used.

THE PREOPERATIVE PERIOD

The majority of patients coming to colectomy are those who have been ill for periods ranging from several months to several years, most commonly with ulcerative colitis, and less often with other inflammatory or, occasionally, neoplastic diseases of the colon. Statistically, these diseases affect individuals younger on the average than those who are to have colostomies. Thus we see students, or young men and women just beginning careers or starting families, afflicted with prolonged, debilitating and expensive illness, hospitalization, and surgery. This age group has the least insurance coverage and lowest financial resources, which are further diminished by recurring episodes of illness, interruption of employment, and sometimes frequent hospitalization. So we begin at this point to consider the psychological drain resulting from concern about material things as well as the continuing threat to health which contributes to the depression of almost all individuals in this group. In addition to worry about the monetary aspects of chronic illness and recurrent unemployability, concern about physical debility and consequent sexual incompetence contribute to this depression. Probably in this stage the ability to perform the sex act as such is not of great concern to the individual, especially during an exacerbation of the disease process, since at these times the patient is primarily attempting to survive. However, each patient is aware that restoration to a reasonably normal pattern of sexual interest and activity is the accepted mode of life in our society at present. Rehabilitation will not be complete if these criteria are not met. Most women anticipate marriage and children as the measure of personal fulfillment and are understandably depressed by the fear that this may be denied them because of their supposed disability and suspected physical unacceptability. Men, though perhaps not as committed to the same pattern as women, are depressed at the anticipation of a condition which they fear may result in sexual as well as physical weakening. In both men and women this fear, and consequent depression is a perfectly normal reaction and is not basically different from other patients. The fear of the unknown affects every intelligent individual facing major surgery.

In this situation however, there are frequently fewer facts made available to the patient than in the case of more common procedures; and this is due to the fact that general surgeons and nurses are not well-informed on these points and retain the idea from years past when complications involving sexual function apparently were prevalent, that difficulties in this area will probably occur.

As will become apparent, the incidence of decrement in sexual function is quite low in males as measured in several parameters by Dlin, Perlman, and Ringold (1969). In women, numerous instances of successfully completed pregnancies by ileostomates are perhaps an indirect measure, but those who responded directly to questionnaire studies indicated no significant decrease in sexual interest or activity following surgery.

If surgeons become aware of these recent studies and the newer prognoses to be expected from improved surgery, they can significantly help to improve the patient's state of mind in the preoperative period. Nevertheless the authors, Fleming (1964) and Druss (1969), of a number of articles mention also the distinct desirability of *preoperative* visits by lay members of the local ileostomy group if one is available. Patients are not rarely hesitant to ask the surgeon about matters pertaining to postoperative sexual adjustment. Experience shows that the patient, seeing an obviously healthy, active, and effective person who is already an ileostomate, who has come particularly to visit him and is not rushed, is encouraged to ask questions about those things which have been bothering him, often including the most intimate details, with less embarrassment than he feels in talking with professionals. Further, the ostomate frequently can answer these questions with more accuracy and detail, drawing upon his own experience, than can the surgeon.

In this preoperative period, the patient's family may be a very powerful positive or negative factor in the patient's psychological adjustment, depending on their reaction to the illness and to the anticipated changes which they fear may be present afterward. They, even more than the patient, are beset by misleading information from well-meaning friends, they have less opportunity to talk with the surgeon perhaps, and their attitude may swing the balance for or against a smooth adjustment. Here too, those other than the surgeon may be able to take the load from his shoulders by counseling the family. The enterostomal therapist may be of considerable help, but at this stage the information required deals with generalities and nontechnical points, and the lay visitor again can relieve the professional staff of this time-consuming but essential task.

There is a relatively small percentage of patients who come to colectomy because of acute ulcerative colitis, without a background of chronic illness, and who therefore may have been spared a long preoperative course of worry, fear, and consequent depression. These patients, however, frequently will have the complications of toxic megacolon; peritonitis; involvement of other organs, such as hepatitis and nephritis; and a depressive state from toxicity alone which may result in disorientation and, at times, frank hallucinations and delusions. Fortunately, these seldom leave any permanent residuals, if successful colectomy can be accomplished. Unfortunately, the deviations from normal contact with reality may be so selective and insidious that in an occasional unfortunate case the patient cannot grasp the possibilities involved, refuses to accept his doctor's advice and will not consent to the necessary surgery, with tragic results.

So we see that the preoperative period is characterized by anxiety and depression greater than is usual for patients anticipating general types of major surgery. The overt activity of the patient in this mood may be characterized by resentment toward others around him and lack of patience, so that the nursing personnel find him uncooperative and demanding. Reassurances frequently fall on deaf ears unless accompanied by some concrete evidence of the probability of a successful outcome of the planned surgery. It is for this reason that it cannot be stated too strongly that unless a patient is too ill to understand, preoperative counseling by an ostomate is of inestimable value. At this time, technical advice about appliances is out of place, except in cases where an elective interval colectomy is planned. Here, the enterostomal therapist, if available, may assist in determining the most suitable site for the stoma, and may actually apply a face plate and pouch to the abdomen in the proper position and allow the patient to wear it for a day. Patients who have had this done report that it has eased the tension greatly to have this experience preoperatively. Obviously, the majority of patients do not approach surgery in circumstances quite this satisfactory; but for the patient who is not too ill to understand, the appearance before him of an individual in obvious good health, active, well-dressed and happy, who has gone through the same experience and achieved the desired end-stage, may very possibly make the difference between a tranquil, receptive patient and one who is despairing and hopeless. The attitude of those surgeons who refuse to permit preoperative contact between an ostomate-visitor and an oriented and coherent patient seems totally without justification from the psychological point of view and contrary to the opinion expressed by every ostomate who was afforded the opportunity to have preoperative counseling.

The contact with the patient's spouse, or in applicable cases the parents, affords an opportunity to further influence for the better the course which the patient will take. These individuals represent almost the only contact the patient still has with his past reality and hope of future normality. Almost everything in the hospital environment is foreign to the patient—the physical surroundings, the personnel, the "sights, sounds, and smells." The amount of time the surgeon spends with the patient is a very small portion of the day and night. All this predisposes and contributes to loss of contact with the patient's reality. If, in addition, those on whom the patient feels he can rely—husband or wife, parents—are unsure of the situation and uninformed about the probable postoperative situation, the patient is placed in an almost untenable situation because the uncertainty of those around him is surely transmitted to him. This is not to suggest that an overly optimistic prognosis should be given to the family, nor that the seriousness of the situation be minimized. However, here again the surgeon may call upon those who have been through this experience to confer with the family, and answer certain nontechnical questions relating to the patient's expected future activities, social acceptance, fitting into the household routine, and so forth. For this specific purpose, some of the ostomy organizations have "non-ostomate counseling services" which are composed of the spouses and parents of ostomates, capable of answering questions relating to these points, and giving reassurance for the future. These people are sufficiently well-informed that they will not usurp the doctor's function of giving specific advice or prognosis, but on a nonprofessional level frequently can answer questions which family members will not or cannot remember to ask the surgeon. This service has proved to be a boon to families, but even more so it is an aid to the surgeon who is thus relieved of time-consuming counseling in nontechnical areas in which he may not be too well-informed.

THE IMMEDIATE POSTOPERATIVE PERIOD

The two or three days immediately after surgery—or longer for very ill patients—are not different from the same period for any patient after a major operative procedure. The patient achieves awareness, and then self-identification and orientation as the effect of postoperative sedatives and narcotics decreases. For those who were more ill preoperatively, with toxic psychotic manifestations, the course may be variable, with hours or even days of nearly normal reaction alternating with recurring disorientation or delusional episodes. But sooner or later the usual psychological reaction appears, and the first stage may be described as a state of grief, or deprivation, in which the patient displays depressive reactions related to the loss of a portion of the body. This reaction is common to all patients who have undergone an amputation resulting in a visible change in the body, requiring a reconstruction of the self-image. This reaction usually does not occur in patients who have undergone equally extensive surgery which does not change a basic physiologic function or body structure visible to the patient. Thus a patient undergoing pneumonectomy, for example, has probably had approximately as extensive a procedure as total colectomy, but still breathes in the same way, though there are some changes perhaps in physical capacity. With the formation of an ileostomy there has been a visible—to the patient at least—change in a physiological function which can never be restored to normal. Secondly, the excreta now appearing uncontrollably represent material which the patient has been taught from childhood is "dirty, untouchable, and usually unmentionable." The strength and persistence of this "taboo" may be demonstrated by the feeling expressed by an ileosomate of several years who states he is completely accustomed to emptying and changing his appliance without any feeling of contamination if the excreta happens to get on the fingers of his right hand, which may occur frequently. But if any of this material accidentally gets on his left hand he feels exactly as he would have before his colectomy, and must immediately scrub the hand well in order to feel clean again.

The grieving reaction which the patient feels at first is gradually supplanted as the patient reconstructs his self-image. This can be helped greatly by affording an opportunity for him to confer again with a successful ileostomate. At this early stage, instruction is still not so important as providing the immediate contact with the "end-result." This stage of the psychological reconstruction, like the other stages, cannot be denied and cannot be rushed. The patient may be helped through it by sympathy and understanding, but if those attending the patient brush it away as unimportant, or fail to support the patient in this area, the further stages will not be achieved so readily, and the patient will lose all rapport with those responsible for restoring him to health.

Though the patient may appear to be, and actually is, quite passive in this period, it is a time of delicate balance in beginning psychological readjustment; and in the empty spaces of the daily hospital routine, the words, the actions, and the attitudes of those attending the patient are grasped at and frequently given much greater importance than the physician or nurse ever intends. Thus the therapist or nurse in the very first few days can set the pattern of the patient's attitude toward his stoma. If the attendant finds it unpleasant to view the stoma, handle the dressings, change the appliance, or to be in the room in which odors can be quite strong at times, this is probably only natural. If the condition were a temporary one, no real harm would be done. But if the patient notices any reaction of this sort he is immediately convinced that he will always offend, and greater harm is done him. An attendant who cannot master his actions and expression under these circumstances should never be permitted to care for any ostomate in the immediate post-operative period.

In this period, then, should begin the instruction in self-care which is absolutely essential to complete rehabilitation. No ilestomate who does not routinely do all that is necessary in this area entirely by himself could be considered rehabilitated. This is not to indicate that a spouse or parent should not be willing and able to take over completely in an emergency since such a plan is wise. An ileostomate of school age or older, unless prevented by some other physical impairment, should not be dependent on any other person for ileostomy management.

In view of the need to begin instruction, and the requirement that the attendant display an undisturbed acceptance of the stoma and all its functions and paraphernalia, the stoma therapist, if available, should personally handle this portion of patient care for the first few days. Since qualified enterostomal therapists are, at this writing, not commonly available in all hospitals, one or more individuals on each shift, competent to attend suitably to this problem, should be trained by, and under the supervision of, the therapist if there be one, or a member of the surgical staff. In this very important period, the patient with a new ileostomy should not be subjected to the ministrations of a well-meaning but uninstructed or unpracticed individual who cannot restrain feelings of disgust to which the patient is so very sensitive, especially since at this time he is himself wavering between this reaction and the hope that others will not be repelled by his new condition. In this period when the patient wants desperately to believe that complete recovery with return to normal interpersonal relationships, self-confidence, and physical competence is now only a short time away, a single unfortunate statement may so severely alter his progress that rehabilitation may be postponed indefinitely, or conceivably not achieved at all.

During these first few days, if there has not been an opportunity to do so preoperatively, the patient is introduced gradually to the appliance and its use. Physical weakness, easy fatigability, and perhaps temporarily dulled mentality from toxicity or drugs require that observation precede application. However, if the attendant is sufficiently experienced to be expert in the practical use of these objects, the patient gains confidence from this alone. If, on the other hand, an attendant obviously does not know which part is which, or what comes next, the patient again despairs.

At this time, further contact with the patient's family by the stoma therapist or ostomy club visitor may save the patient and the family much strain. The patient, still uncertain of the outcome, or weary with the struggle and the great physical weakness, may berate family members, or make unreasonable demands. If the family realizes that this is the usual outward manifestation of the grief reaction, and that the patient must be helped to work his way through it as a part of the recovery process, they can more readily accept vagaries of the patient's reactions, and the recovery period is made smoother for all

It seems obvious that the psychological aspects of patient care in this first few days after surgery involve more sensitivity to disturbance and yet are more important to the goal of complete rehabilitation than in any other similar time period. No specific length of time can be assigned to this phase of grief changing slowly into acceptance, since the physical and mental recovery rate of patients, as well as their basic mentality and dexterity before the onset of the illness, vary widely. A few patients, notably those who undergo interval colectomy, with a high level of intelligence and dexterity as their norm, may be quite well adjusted and able to undertake total self care within ten to fifteen days postoperatively. Many others may not achieve this level in less than a year, if ever. In this period, then, the selection of personnel attending the patient is more important than at any other time. Visitors also should be screened so that well-meaning but ill-informed friends or even members of the immediate family are not permitted to disrupt the patient's early phases of personality reconstruction by ill-timed or thoughtless remarks or questions. The patient must learn to feel secure in his own identity and competence before being forced to explain or defend a condition he is only beginning to understand and accept.

In this area more time—specifically the number of minutes and hours—is required to answer all the patient's questions as he learns to ask them, and those of the family as they perceive the possibilities involved in ileostomy care, if both patient and relatives are to feel satisfied and not "brushed-off," than the attending surgeon has to give. The enterostomal therapist is the logical second choice, and indeed in these situations in which a general surgeon may do only one or two ileostomy procedures a year, the enterostomal therapist may be better qualified than the surgeon to answer questions as to appliances, diet, hygiene, skin care, and social contacts. In fact, an experienced lay member of the local ostomy club can be called upon for socioeconomic guidance, and thus release both surgeon and enterostomal therapist for the more technical and specialized care of other patients. Not infrequently the patient, and even more often, family members will find it easier to ask questions in this area of the visiting ostomate than the professional, because they identify themselves and their level of knowledge more easily with the lay person. As all doctors are aware, there are some people who hesitate to ask questions about those things which concern them most, fearing to "bother" the doctor, or "take too much time." And some doctors, perhaps unconsciously, foster this attitude because of the pressure of time or an unawareness of the emotional state of patient and family.

Nevertheless, it is in the immediate postoperative period that the pattern of acceptance of the ileostomy, willingness to learn how best to cope with it, and determination to overcome obstacles and achieve complete rehabilitation begin.

THE IMMEDIATE POST-HOSPITAL PERIOD

When the patient has left the hospital and is dependent on his own resources for ileostomy care, he first becomes truly concerned about his future role in society. Certainly he has given it much thought before this, but in the protective situation of hospital care it has been somewhat impersonal. Now, even though he knows that technical help is quickly available for medical problems, he must orient himself to his own environment, and adjust his requirements to whatever is available to him, or alter them as is necessary or possible. Among the many aspects involved in this will be his relationship to his spouse if he is married, or the possibilities of future marriage if he is not. After any prolonged or severe illness, or extensive surgical procedure, the ability to engage in normal sexual activity, or indeed to develop a normal interest in these matters, is slow to return to normal. In the time between the restoration of interest and that of performance, many males will become very concerned, having perhaps been told, or suspecting, that surgery done in such close proximity to the genitalia might have some permanent deleterious effect. Indeed, judging from the prevalence of this idea it may be that in the early years of abdominoperincal resection, such effects might have been common. Now, the percentage of men reporting permanent changes in these functions—not impotence but definite decrease in sexual activity —is only 15 percent. The great majority of males, when physical rehabilitation has restored them to approximate pre-surgery or pre-illness levels, find their patterns of sexual activity unchanged. That is, those whose interests were strong in this area generally found themselves following the same patterns. Those whose social and sexual activities were previously of minor importance found them about the same after return to normal.

Female ileostomates are usually less concerned with sexual performance and much more with the possibility that the stoma and associated paraphernalia will make them physically less attractive, and the younger age groups are fearful that the extensive surgery will interfere with childbearing. It has been quite well established now that fertility, pregnancy, and normal delivery are seldom interfered with by the presence of the ileostomy, and conversely that pregnancy seldom produces complications in the care and function of the stoma. Many ostomates have married, become pregnant, and delivered normally without any special care or restrictions. The question of whether the stoma decreases the acceptability of the female to her partner is so dependent on the ostomate's own feeling about it, and that of the spouse, that no generalities can be made. Various authors who have worked with quite large groups of ostomates through questionnaires report many marriages of women who have ileostomies, with no greater incidence of divorce or separation than the average for all marriages. Some young female ostomates seem firmly convinced that marriage is impossible for them, but investigations in depth suggests that the stoma may receive the blame for a temperament more suited to the single life even before the illness began.

In the immediate post-hospital period, the adjustment to total self-care of the stoma is based on effective and knowledgeable education in the hospital, pursued in the home environment by further assistance from the enterostomal therapist if this is possible, and by a close follow-up by the local ileostomates. This is accomplished where possible by drawing the patient into a group of people who have adjusted successfully to life with a stoma. These groups can provide the patient with on-going contact with new developments in appliances and their uses, and can initiate social relationships with a group to which he need make no explanations or apologies. By no means all, or even a majority, of ileostomates will or should remain active in such a group indefinitely. Probably the majority, as they approach total rehabilitation, will become inactive as far as attending meetings or other club activities. Fortunately, there will always be a few who recognize the help they received from such a group during their own periods of illness, and who will feel that they in turn can repay the debt by visiting and instructing new ostomates. However, if an individual is depressed by continuing association with these people, he should not feel obligated to remain active.

THE END RESULT OF REHABILITATION

The consensus of opinion among the rather small number of authors who have studied the psychosexual status of ostomates seems to be that the final rehabilitation of the ostomate to a position in his family and community which represents the maximum recovery for him—it may be different from that which he formerly occupied—is the product of several elements. These elements include the basic psychological, and to some extent physical, structure which he brings to the crisis of colectomy; secondly, the manner of presenting the ultimatum of surgery to him and to his family and gaining their understanding and cooperation in all the complex facets of ileostomy management; thirdly, his ability to accept, at first passively and then actively, the structural and functional changes which have been thrust upon him, and lastly his ability to create a self-image in the new situation which permits him to develop the self-confidence and emotional stability necessary to again engage in all those activities which were normal and desirable for him in the pre-illness state.

In the first area, the basic psychosexual condition of the patient who will become an ileostomate, statistical analyses have shown him to be, on the average, a person in the productive and family-oriented years, usually with above average education, income potential, and perhaps intelligence. But not infrequently he is also a person having had some psychological problems which in some cases have required professional help. In the second area, the illness itself is usually accompanied by psychological as well as physical changes, at times quite profound; and in this period and for some time thereafter there is less regard for matters pertaining to sex than those involved with survival itself. In this period the manner in which the prospect of ileostomy is presented to the patient is vital, and it is almost universally stated by patients, and now more frequently by surgeons too, that contact with a successful ileostomate frequently makes the difference between calm acceptance and frank despair, or even flat refusal to undergo surgery. It is at this point that a potential ileostomate may listen to reassuring words by doctors, nurses, even family members, about the necessity of surgery to effect a cure, and how it is quite possible to live a normal life with a stoma. But consciously or not, the patient looks at these people who do not have a stoma, and reassurances are weakened. If an ostomate appears and can say the same thing, it becomes believable. Here also the understanding of the family of what an ileostomate is and does is of help to them and thus to the patient, and obviously to the surgeon and professional staff.

In the third stage, the immediate postoperative period, trained and knowledgeable care of the stoma is the most heartening experience to the patient in his passive state. With increasing personal involvement in its care, under expert guidance, the patient is assisted in rebuilding a satisfactory self-image with a minimum of concern about the future. Only if instruction and practice in self-care are afforded by the surgeon himself if he has sufficient time and experience, or by a competent person such as the enterostomal therapist, can the ostomate begin with confidence to achieve the self-sufficiency which is absolutely essential to total rehabilitation.

In the fourth and final stage, surgeon and enterostomal therapist are left behind, though always readily available in case of complications, and the ostomate must progress under his own power. The family is the greatest factor for—or against—success, and most ostomates who do well are aware of this. The most successful ones are those whose spouses, in particular, and other family members as well, as willing and prepared to accept the changes and to treat the ostomate as a whole person, without disability, able to live a full and normal life without significant restriction or special requirements. In this fully rehabilitated state sexual interest and activity are usually unchanged from the pre-illness norm for that individual. For those ostomates who had personality defects before illness, colectomy seldom affords a cure of the defect. Also, a small percentage may have recurring complications serious enough to require further hospitalization or surgery, and a moderate number will have minor complications. For the great majority, however, life with an ostomy is so much better than continuing illness, that very few would choose any possible alternative. The importance of the psychological aspects of both this illness and its "cure" must not be overlooked, and all available resources should be known and made available to the patient and his family to achieve the fully rehabilitated ileostomate.

Chapter 5

CASE STUDIES OF SERVICES TO CLIENTS

IN STATE-FEDERAL AGENCIES OF

VOCATIONAL REHABILITATION

CASE OF MR. L. C.

MR. L. C. IS A 51-year-old white male, is married and has three children.

Mr. L. C.'s major disability stems from a total laryngectomy which was performed in May, 1973. The client was in need of an artificial larnyx and speech therapy to restore oral communication. The client cannot perform his chosen occupation without oral communication.

Referral Source

Mr. L. C. was referred for rehabilitation services by the general hospital. The client underwent a laryngectomy in May previous to his referral in July.

Social Data

The client is a member of a strong, cohesive family unit. His family has rallied around and given him great support and encouragement.

The client had been a manager for a chain grocery store and can return to that position after physical restoration.

Psychological Data

Psychological testing was not deemed appropriate in this case since the client wishes to, and has the intellectual ability to, return to his former employment. His position is being held open for him by his employer.

The client applied for services and has cooperated in every way possible. However, the client's morale must be maintained through this period of adjustment and uncertainty. Counseling and guidance will be provided. The client also receives much encouragement and support from his wife and children.

Medical Information

Other than the squamous cell carcinoma of the larynx, the client was in good physical condition. He had been hospitalized biefly in 1964 for colitis with no recurrence.

Mr. L. C. underwent a total laryngectomy in May, 1973 and has apparently recovered from surgery nicely. Upon referral to the Bureau of Rehabilitation Service (BRS), the client was judged ready for speech therapy and restoration of oral communication.

Vocational and Educational History, Financial Situation, Cost of Case

Other than the client's experience as a chain grocery store manager, no additional vocational or educational background information was provided.

The client's financial situation had deteriorated because of his illness. Although the client's income level had been much higher than BRS usually helps, his level of living was geared to full income and he had been on sick leave at one-half pay for over a year. He had exhausted all savings and resources. No figures were given as to the client's monthly income.

The cost of this case to BRS amounted to $502, broken down as follows: prosthetic appliance (Electrolarynx) $350; speech therapy, $152. The American Cancer Society contributed equally ($152) to the cost of therapy.

Services Provided

Rehabilitation provided the client with the electrolarynx and the necessary speech therapy. In addition the client and his family received counseling and guidance.

Summary

This case is still astir and in the follow-up stage. All indications are that this person will be successfully rehabilitated in the near future.

CASE OF MISS D. M.

Miss D. M. is a 47-year-old, black, unmarried female. No information was given as to her educational level.

Major disability was diagnosed as a uterine fibroid tumor requiring a hysterectomy.

Referral Source

Miss D. M. was referred for vocational rehabilitation services by the Family Health Clinic. The client is employed by the Clinic full-time. Because the client had no financial resources to pay for corrective surgery and because she would have been unable to continue in her job without the required surgery, the client was accepted for rehabilitative services.

Social Data

Miss D. M. lives alone. The Family Health Clinic is a part of the Model Cities Program for the community. The client's position there is that of a home aid worker assigned to taking care of elderly persons. Staff at the center are pleased with the client's work and all indications are that this is a suitable placement.

Miss D. M. will depend on friends to assist in providing for her needs while she recovers from surgery.

Psychological Data

No psychological data were given in the file.

Medical Information

No medical reports were included in the file material. The counselor stated that corrective surgery was successful, enabling the client to return to full-time competitive employment.

Vocational History, Educational History, Brief
Financial Situation, Cost of Case

Vocational and educational background data are absent from the file. The client had no financial resources to pay for corrective surgery. Her salary as a home aid worker was $280.00 a month. She had no other income or resources.

The cost of the case to BRS amounted to $794.14; broken down as follows: hysterectomy surgery, $250; anesthesia, $49.50; hospitalization, $494.64.

Services Provided

In addition to the above expenses paid by BRS, the client was to receive biweekly contact from the counselor following surgery to assure that she was physically restored and able to resume her employment. The only evidence of follow-up was once in May and once more in August.

Summary

This case closed as a successful status 26 (rehabilitated) as the client made a complete recovery and returned to her work.

CASE OF MR. J. P.

Mr. J. P., a white male, age thirty-eight, is married with two dependents, and completed the first five grades of schooling.

Major disability results from cancer of the mandible. Reconstruction surgery is necessary for functioning purposes. Mr. J. P. has been unemployed due to this physical condition.

Referral Source

Mr. J. P. was referred for rehabilitative services by the local general hospital in January, 1973, approximately four years after undergoing cancer surgery.

Social Data

No social data was given, except a brief discussion of educational and vocational history.

The client had previously been employed as a mechanic. It was felt that because of this work experience and his limited educational background, an appropriate vocational objective would be for him to return to this line of employment.

Psychological Data

No discussion of the psychological aspects were found in the file. It was briefly mentioned that the client was eager to cooperate in a program of physical restoration and was anxious to seek employment as a mechanic.

The counselor also mentioned that the client would be aided with any problems that he might encounter during physical restoration and later in adjusting to suitable employment.

Medical Information

Mr. J. P. underwent surgery for the removal of a malignant tumor of the mandible in November 1968. This consisted of removal of the anterior portion of the mandible.

After referral to BRS in January, 1973, the client was supplied with a mandibular splint used in reconstruction surgery.

Vocational and Educational History, Financial Situation, Cost of Case

Vocational and educational background, were previously discussed. In reference to the client's financial situation, his chief means of support was through state aid. The client's monthly income was less than $150.

The cost of this case to BRS was limited to supplying the mandibular splint used in the reconstruction surgery in the amount of $100.

Services Provided

The Bureau of Rehabilitation supplied the mandibular splint and assisted in placement. The client returned to work as a mechanic and is now able to earn $45 per week.

Summary

The reconstruction surgery was successful, and placement was made. The counselor indicated he would "keep in touch with the client in order to insure that this employment remains feasible."

CASE OF MRS. M. R.

Mrs. M. R. is a black female, age fifty, married, and has two dependent children.

Mrs. M. R. required surgery for the removal of a possible carcinoma of the right breast. A radical mastectomy was performed in September, 1972.

Referral Source

The referral source was not named in the file. The referral was made for assistance with surgical expenses to remove the disabling condition which had developed in her right breast.

Social Data

Mrs. M. R. is obviously a person who accepts responsibility. She has raised her family and continues to make a home for her husband and two children. No other information given.

Psychological Data

Because she enjoys her work as a domestic and plans to return to that line of work, psychological testing was not judged necessary.

Medical Information

With the exception of the carcinoma, the client was in good general health. Her doctors expected that within six weeks of surgery, she would be able to return to a full, normal routine. She gave a history of hypertension for six months prior to surgery.

Vocational and Educational History, Financial Situation, Cost of Case

The client had worked for the same family, two days per week as a domestic maid for eleven years. This was her chosen work. She was experienced; the position remained open for her return. No placement services were indicated. No educational background information was available.

There was very little in the file concerning the client's income. She worked two days per week but her income was only $17. No mention was made of her husband's income, if any. The file did state that the family was not on any public assistance roles.

The total cost of services to BRS amounted to $1,000.70, broken down as follows: surgery, $300; biopsy, $50; anesthesia, $93.50; hospitalization, $557.20.

Services Provided

Mrs. M. R. received the above medical services paid for by BRS and also received counseling and guidance during the adjustment period as needed.

Summary

The case was closed in December, 1972 as successful. The client had returned to her former employment and no further services were indicated.

CASE OF MR. H. T.

Mr. H. T., white male, age forty-one, is married and has two dependent children.

The client had been rendered 100 percent disabled as a result of surgery performed in August, 1972. The client suffered from metastatic squamous cell carcinoma of the mandibular area bilaterally. Surgery consisted of a right, radical neck mandibulectomy. In September, 1972 some reconstruction of the upper lip was performed. Mr. H. T. presented severe facial deformity secondary to surgery. The client could not speak and was very reserved around strangers. Also, exposure to people increased the chance of infection in the surgical site.

Referral Source

Mr. H. T. was referred for rehabilitative services by the Social Security Administration. The client was 100 percent disabled and in need of reconstruction of the mandible in the nature of bone grafts. Tracheostomy and feeding tubes were still in place.

Social Data

As stated, the client is married with two dependent children. The family was in a state of financial stress. Their savings had been exhausted in the attempt to meet medical bills not covered by insurance. The client's wife couldn't work because she constantly had to care for the client and the children.

The client had been an assistant manager for a railway company and all indications were that his job was being held open and would be restored when he was physically able to return to work.

Psychological Data

Psychological testing was not felt to be necessary, as the client hoped to return to his former employment, for which he had previously been well suited.

Because of the gross facial deformity and the inability to communicate orally, the client had become very reserved, avoiding people. The client could not actually meet with the counselor because exposure to people heightened the prospect of introducing infection. Also, prior to this present illness and disability, the client had been financially stable. The surgery and unemployment had drained the family financially thus creating additional emotional problems. Guidance and counseling were indicated for both the client and the family.

Medical Information

The client had an uneventful medical background until he sought medical assistance in July, 1972. The client presented a mass of the right chin and jaw, with a duration of approximately two years. When he came to BRS, the cancer surgery and initial reconstruction surgery had been completed. Still necessary was the bulk of reconstruction in the form of bone grafts to reconstruct the mandible, rotation flops, and the lower lip.

Vocational and Educational History, Financial
Situation, Cost of Case

As stated, the client had been an assistant manager for a

railway company. He had held this position for four years prior to surgery. Because of a favorable medical prognosis and the railway company's expressed wish for the client to return to his former job, it was feasible to consider this.

The client's educational background was not discussed.

The client's financial situation was drastic. He was receiving social security disability benefits; however, the family had no resources left with which to pay the medical bills. The client's medical benefits had been exhausted. In addition, a large part of the family's meager income had gone each week for special diet foods and medication for the client. The available income for the family of four is approximately $350 monthly.

The cost of the case to rehabilitative services amounted to $3,440.24, broken down as follows: reconstruction surgery $1,500; anesthesia, $195; hospitalization, $1,745.24.

Services Provided

In addition to reconstruction surgery, guidance and counseling concerned the emotional needs of the client and his family. Assistance in working out the best way possible of the extreme financial burden.

Summary

Follow-up consisting of close contact with physician and family is actively being conducted at this writing. When the client's period of isolation is over, assistance will be given in adjustment to employment once again.

CASE OF MRS. O. R.

Mrs. O. R. is a white female, age fifty-four, is married and has no dependent children. She has an eighth-grade education.

Mrs. O. R.'s major disability was a feminine disorder resulting from pelvic inflammatory disorder (cancer of the uterus). Her condition caused her much pain, soreness, excessive bleeding and had weakened her to the point that she was no longer able to care for her home and disabled husband.

Referral Source

The client was referred for rehabilitation service by David K., a surgeon. Due to the client's condition, she was in need of a hysterectomy. The prognosis was excellent that following corrective surgery, the client would be able to resume her home-making duties.

Social Data

There are five members in this family. The client's husband is disabled because of black lung. The client takes care of her husband and keeps house. Mrs. O. R. has no income of her own and the only source of income is her husband's monthly check for black lung.

Psychological Factors

Psychological testing was not felt appropriate because the client's vocational objective was to return to housekeeping duties following corrective surgery.

It was mentioned in the reports that the client was cooperative. She was to receive counseling and guidance in regard to her postoperative care and treatment.

Medical Information

Mrs. O. R. is an obese lady of fifty-four years. The need for the hysterectomy restricted her physical activities. The prognosis was excellent for recovery after surgery. No previous medical history was available.

Vocational and Educational History, Financial Situation, Cost of Case

It was mentioned that the client did not progress beyond the eighth grade. No vocational background information was available.

With only the disability benefits from her husband's black lung as a source of income, the family was limited to less than $300 per month. The client was not receiving public assistance.

The cost of the case to BRS amounted to $360, broken down as follows: surgery, $300; anesthesia, $60.

The client had some medical insurance to cover hospitalization.

Services Provided

Services included corrective surgery plus counseling and guidance.

Summary

This case was a successful closure in status 26 (rehabilitated). The client made the necessary physical and mental adjustments following corrective surgery.

CASE OF MR. W. A.

Mr. W. A. is a 54-year-old white male, divorced, living alone in an apartment. He supports a sixteen-year-old daughter who lives with her mother. He has two sons ages nineteen and twenty who are independent and self-supporting.

Mr. W. A.'s disability stems from multiple lymph node enlargement in various parts of the body which requires surgery and hospitalization.

Referral Source

Mr. W. A. was referred to Vocational Rehabilitation in January, 1973 for rehabilitative services by his physician who recommended hospitalization and surgery.

Social Data

The client is a carpenter by trade and will function as one following corrective surgery. No other social information was discussed.

Psychological Data

Because the client planned on returning to his previous vocation—carpentry finisher—no psychological testing was felt appropriate. Other than the indication of counseling and guidance, no other psychological information was discussed.

Medical Information

No background medical information was provided in the file. The absence of medical reports was also obvious. The type of cancer the client suffered is very dangerous and progressive. Surgery and medication were necessary to arrest the progress of the disease.

Vocational and Educational History, Financial Situation, Cost of Case

No educational or vocational background information was discussed in the file other than, of course, mentioning the client's chosen occupation. Following treatment, the client did return to work as a carpentry finisher.

The client was not on public assistance roles. His total monthly earnings amounted to an average of $300 to $325 when he was working. Although living alone, he supports his sixteen-year-old daughter.

The total cost of the case to rehabilitation services amounted to $398.16 including surgery, biopsy, anesthesia, and hospitalization.

Services Provided

After medical treatment, the client became less cooperative in keeping counseling appointments. He stated he was reluctant to keep appointments because he felt able to proceed on his own.

Summary

The case was closed as a successful status 26 (rehabilitated). Follow-up was not indicated as the client was reluctant to keep appointments.

APPENDIX

IN ORDER TO understand the counseling and rehabilitation process in working with the cancer patient one should be able to review a detailed case study and answer the questions below. The answers to these questions should be developed in order to demonstrate the breadth of concern of rehabilitation counselors in working with the cancer patient. Cancer presents a very complex system of problems with which the rehabilitation team must deal. These include generally medical, psychological, vocational, social and marital problems. We would suggest the individual interested in being better equipped to counsel and rehabilitate the cancer patient should review detailed case studies and respond to the following questions:

1. What are the special problems of rehabilitation of the individual with cancer?
   a. medical
   b. psychological
   c. social
   d. vocational
   e. other
2. What counseling services might appropriately be provided?
   a. vocational
   b. personal
   c. educational
   d. other
3. What additional services should have been offered or could have been offered?
   a. medical
   b. other psychological
   c. other social
4. Was the individual with cancer eligible for vocational

rehabilitation services through the state agency? Yes......
No...... On what basis?

5. What type of diagnostic information was needed in order to evaluate the vocational plan?

6. How was the vocational objective decided in this case?

7. Could this person's problems been dealt with differently—to improve services to him—what would you have done?

8. How were the services of other professionals, including psychologists, physicians, occupational therapists, etc. coordinated by the counselor?

9. Did other professional persons understand what the counselor really needed from them in order to help the client?

10. Was there documented reporting back to other involved professional team workers?

11. Was the case recorded adequately? Yes...... No......
Why?......

12. Was the client involved in all decision making?

13. What were the client's real concerns? Did he really get the services he wanted?

14. What were the concerns of the counselor?

15. Were there adequate follow-along services?

16. Are social and rehabilitation services in your state less than adequate, adequate, or more than adequate for this disability group? How? Why?

17. How would the client evaluate rehabilitation services?

18. What other questions should be asked in order to evaluate rehabilitation services to the client?

INDEX

143

Preoperative counseling, 118
Postoperative disfigurement
    psychological reaction, 54-55
Preoperative radiotherapy, 43
Presidents' Commission on Heart
    Disease, Cancer and Stroke, 21
Presurgical management, 104
Prognosis, 9
Prosthesis, 61, 65
Prosthetic appliance, 131
Pseudolarynx, 56
Psychiatric referral, 103
Psychiatrist, 47, 55
Psychoanalysis, 80
Psychoanalytic therapy, 76
Psychodynamic material, 100
Psychological
    adjustment, 117
    readjustment, 121
    reconstruction, 121
    services, 53
    stress, 59
    testing, 130
Psychologist, 37, 47, 55, 66
Psychosexual condition, 127
Psychotherapeutic communication, 105
Psychotherapeutic measures, 70
Psychotherapeutic methods, 100
Psychotherapy, 70, 76, 79, 96
    theory, 69

Q

"Quality of Survival of the Cancer
    Patient," 25

R

Radiation, 8, 104
Radical mastectomy, 64, 134
Radical surgery, 44
Radioactive iodine, 45
Radioresistant tumor, 41
Radiosensitivity, 41
Radiotherapist, 37, 39
Radiotherapy, 38, 39, 41, 57

preoperative, 43
Rapport, 76
Reassurance, 85
Reconstruction surgery, 132, 136
Regional chemotherapy, 42
Regional Maxillofacial Restoration
    Center, 65
Rehabilitation
    adjustment, 12
    counselor, 14, 25, 37, 47, 61, 62, 66
    eligibility policies, 65
    potential, 5
    program, 9
    services, 6, 63
Rehabilitation Record, 22
Remissions, 46
Renneker, R., 104, 114
Resentment, 77
Retinoblastomas, 42
Rusk, Howard, 23, 64
Rynearson, E., 114

S

Samuelson, Cecil O., ix, 3
Samuelson, Kent Mitchell, ix, 3
Sarcoma, 7
Selective attention, 81, 82
Self-concept, 59
Self-image, 121
Separation trauma, 48
Sheltered work situation, 27
Shimkin, Michael B., 9, 23
Simon, A. J., 113
Social adjustment, 18
Social Security disability benefits, 137
Social unacceptability, 59
Social worker, 47, 55, 66
Somatic delusion, 102
Somatic reactions, 71
Speech
    esophageal, 55-56
    therapy, 129-131
Stehlin, John S., Jr., 39, 46-48
Stoma, 122
    therapist, 123
Superego action, 96

DATE D